T0191878

Pediatric Continuous Renal Replacement Therapy

Farahnak Assadi • Fatemeh Ghane Sharbaf

Pediatric Continuous Renal Replacement Therapy

Principles and Practice

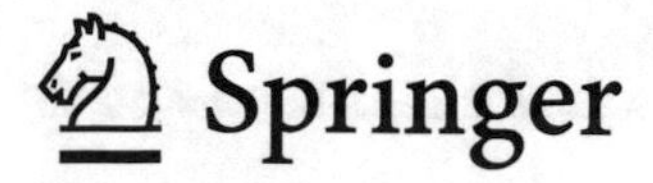

Farahnak Assadi, M.D.
Professor Emeritus
Department of Pediatrics
Section of Nephrology
Rush University Medical Center
Chicago, IL, USA

Fatemeh Ghane Sharbaf, M.D.
Associate Professor
Department of Pediatrics
Section of Nephrology
Mashhad University of Medical Sciences
Mashhad, Iran

ISBN 978-3-319-79905-6 ISBN 978-3-319-26202-4 (eBook)
DOI 10.1007/978-3-319-26202-4

Springer Cham Heidelberg New York Dordrecht London

Softcover re-print of the Hardcover 1st edition 2016

Printed on acid-free paper

Springer International Publishing AG Switzerland is part of Springer Science+Business Media (www.springer.com)

This book is dedicated to all patients for whom we care and always teach us so much.

Preface

Acute kidney injury (AKI) is a common cause of morbidity and mortality rates in critically ill patients requiring intensive care therapies (40–50 %). The incidence of AKI varies from 5 % of all hospitalized patients to 30–40 % of patients admitted to the pediatric intensive care unit. The critically ill children with AKI often have multiple organ dysfunctions and are frequently treated with several drugs including antibiotics, anticonvulsants, vasopressors, and antihypertensive and cardiovascular agents or which require appropriate dosing and interval. Despite significant improvements in the care of critically ill patients, the mortality and morbidity associated with AKI remains high (>50 %) and can lead to end-stage renal disease.

Approach to the treatment of AKI patients requiring dialysis has gone under evolution with the advent of continuous renal replacement therapy (CRRT) techniques over the last two decades. Critically ill and hemodynamic instable children better tolerate CRRT than the intermittent hemodialysis. CRRT technology attempts to replace the excretory function of the kidney. CRRT provides a slow and gentle fluid removal from body much like the native kidneys and removes inflammatory mediators of sepsis such as interleukin, TNF-alpha, and complement. CRRT also provides adequate nutritional support for the catabolic AKI patients, a controlled desired fluid balance.

Many AKI patients receiving CRRT suffer from multiple organ dysfunctions and have various types of medications including antibiotics, anticonvulsants, anticoagulants, and cardiovascular agents. Drugs predominantly eliminated by the normal kidneys often undergo substantial changes by CRRT. Therefore, a dose adjustment is required to prevent under dosing of the medication or drug toxicity.

Unfortunately, few clinical studies have been published, and few drugs have been studied pharmacoclinically in intensive care patients. Many guidelines for drug dosing during CRRT are extrapolated from experiences with adult chronic hemodialysis, and there has been a relative paucity of published data about drug dosing during CRRT in critically ill children. Doses used in adults CRRT cannot be directly applied to these children, as the CRRT dialysate prescription and pharmacokinetics are different in adults compared with children. Failure to correctly dose may result in either drug toxicity or treatment failure. In order to understand the optimal drug dosing for children receiving CRRT, one must understand the pattern of water and solutes transport through a semipermeable membrane by all forms of CRRT.

In this book, we review the current understanding of CRRT techniques, with a focus on drug dosing in critically ill children receiving CRRT. The effect of CRRT on drug pharmacokinetics, which provides guidelines whether or not dose adjustment is required, is provided in an accompanying reference table. Variations in the drug properties regarding their molecular weights, dialysis and blood flow rates, and dialysis membranes are discussed. The book also provides a simple and easy method for estimating drug clearance as a function of total creatinine clearance when the information on the pharmacokinetics of a particular drug is not available.

In this book, we provide a series of challenging, clinically oriented case studies. The selected case reports focus on the essential aspects of the patient's presentation and laboratory data and management to accelerate recovery. A series of logical questioning from the presentation is followed by a detailed explanation that reviews recent publications and translates emerging areas of science into data that is useful at the bedside.

We hope that the book will expand the clinical knowledge of nephrology and critical care trainees and other practicing physicians from different specialties who are frequently involved in the care of critically ill children suffering from severe AKI to improve and sustain their quality of life.

We are grateful to the staff at Springer Publishers, Inc., for their outstanding editorial contributions to this endeavor and all those who have dedicated their skills to make this effort entirely possible.

Chicago, IL, USA — Farahnak Assadi
Mashhad, Iran — Fatemeh Ghane Sharbaf

Contents

Abbreviations

ACD	Acid citrate dextrose
ACE	Angiotensin-converting enzyme
ACT	Activated clotting time
ARF	Acute renal failure
AKI	Acute kidney injury
ARDS	Acute respiratory distress syndrome
APPT	Activated partial thromboplastin time
BP	Blood pressure
BUN	Blood urea nitrogen
CL	Clearance
CKD	Chronic kidney disease
Cr	Creatinine
CRRT	Continuous renal replacement therapy
CVVH	Continuous veno-venous replacement therapy
CVVHD	Continuous veno-venous hemodialysis
CVVHDF	Continuous veno-venous hemodiafiltration
ECV	Extracorporeal volume
ESRD	End-stage renal failure
GFR	Glomerular filtration rate
HD	Hemodialysis
HF	Hemofiltration
HIT	Heparin-induced thrombocytopenia
ICU	Intensive care unit
IHD	Intermittent hemodialysis
IJV	Internal jugular vein
INR	International normalization ratio
LMW	Low molecular weight
MODS	Multiple-organ dysfunction syndrome
NSAID	Nonsteroidal anti-inflammatory drug
PD	Peritoneal dialysis
PICU	Pediatric intensive care unit

PK	Pharmacokinetics
PT	Prothrombin time
RCA	Regional citrate anticoagulation
RIFLE	Risk, injury, failure, loss, end-stage kidney disease
RRT	Renal replacement therapy
RVU	Relative unit value
SC	Sieving coefficient
SCUF	Slow continuous ultrafiltration
SIRS	Systemic inflammatory response syndrome
$T_{1/2}$	Half-life
TMP	Transmembrane pressure
TPN	Total parenteral nutrition
UF	Ultrafiltration
V_d	Volume distribution

Chapter 1
Introduction: Acute Kidney Injury and Continuous Renal Replacement Therapy

Introduction

Acute kidney injury (AKI) is a common problem in hospitalized patients and is associated with significant mortality and morbidity [1–5, 8–12, 14, 16, 17, 19–23, 25, 31, 32, 34, 39]. It occurs in 5 % of all hospitalized patients and up to 30 % of critically ill patients [1, 4, 8, 11, 18, 25, 30, 38]. The morbidity and mortality rates are 40 % and 60 %, respectively, in all patients admitted to the pediatric intensive care unit (ICU) [6, 14, 31, 32, 35, 36].

The preponderance of evidence supports the causal link between AKI and subsequent chronic kidney disease (CKD). Unlike a large proportion of adults who develop AKI superimposed on a substrate of hypertension, diabetes mellitus, chronic vascular disease, and underlying CKD, these factors generally do not underlie the development of AKI in children. Thus, the subsequent development of CKD in children surviving an episode of AKI is more readily attributable to residual kidney injury for the AKI.

Severe acute renal injury (AKI) necessitating renal replacement therapy often occurs in a significant proportion of critically ill patients, including patients with septic shock and multiorgan failure [21, 24, 27, 30, 31]. The critically ill and hemodynamic instable children with AKI are frequently treated with continuous renal replacement therapy (CRRT) [6, 7, 10, 13, 26, 27, 33]. CRRT, unlike the traditional hemodialysis and peritoneal dialysis, provides a slow and gentle fluid removal from body much like the native kidneys and removes inflammatory mediators of sepsis such as interleukin, TNF-alpha, and complement [6, 7, 10, 13, 24, 26, 27, 33, 37]. CRRT also provides adequate nutritional support for the catabolic AKI patients and for a controlled desired fluid balance [20].

Underdiagnosed and untreated AKI may lead to CKD and end-stage renal disease. The incidence of CKD and end-stage renal disease has nearly doubled over the last two decades across the globe. With annual mortality for patients on dialysis in the range of 20 %, more people die with treated uremia than with any cancer, except

F. Assadi, F.G. Sharbaf, *Pediatric Continuous Renal Replacement Therapy*,
DOI 10.1007/978-3-319-26202-4_1

for lung cancer. If current trends continue, the toll of end-stage renal disease will exceed that of lung cancer. The burden of disease is paralleled by the enormous cost for delivering end-stage renal disease care [3, 14].

CRRT has become the preferred choice for blood purification and volume control in critically ill children [6, 7, 10, 13, 24, 26, 27, 33, 37]. The reported overall survival rate for children with severe AKI requiring CRRT is 60 % and mortality in infants is comparable with that of older children and adolescents [8, 15, 18, 22, 30].

CRRT treatments have undergone considerable evolution with the advent of new technologies over the last decade [28, 29].

CRRT is indicated in the pediatric population for acute renal failure (AKI), electrolyte abnormalities, catabolic patients with increased nutritional needs, patients with sepsis, poisoning (occasionally in combination with hemodialysis, inborn errors of metabolism, diuretic unresponsive hypervolemia, and hepatic or drug-induced coma) [6, 7, 13, 27, 34, 37]. Additionally, CRRT in conjunction with other therapies such as extracorporeal membranous oxygenation (ECMO), patients with cardiomyopathy on a left-ventricular assist device (LVAD), and the newer hepatic support therapies has also proven to be quite useful [9, 33]. A child with AKI and fluid overload with hemodynamic compromise is a common scenario that many of us would also consider a good candidate. The use of CRRT for inborn error of metabolism is less efficient then hemodialysis yet has been shown to be effective [6].

Several controversies, however, exist over which approach to patient care is most desirable and which form of CRRT should be utilized to achieve the best possible outcome. There are also controversies with respect to what should be the indications for starting such therapy, what is the preferred vascular access, and what kind of anticoagulation should be used. There is also uncertainty with respect to what membranes and filters are preferable and what machines are most appropriate for the patient needs.

While the basic principles of CRRT are similar for adults and children, the application of these modalities in children requires recognition of the unique properties of pediatric hemofiltration. Specific attention to detail, such as extracorporeal blood volume/blood priming (especially in patients <10 kg), nutritional issues, etiological differences in disease processes (i.e., inborn errors of metabolism), access, and line/membrane choice, must be given when dealing with problems in this population [6, 7, 10, 26–29, 37].

References of Section Introduction

1. Andreoli SP. Acute renal failure. Curr Opin Pediatr. 2002;14:183–8.
2. Andreoli SP. Acute renal failure in the newborn. Semin Perinatol. 2004;28(2):112–23.
3. Assadi F. Strategies to reduce the incident of chronic kidney disease in children: time to change. J Nephrol. 2012;26:41–7.
4. Bagshaw SM. Epidemiology of renal recovery after acute renal failure. Curr Opin Crit Care. 2006;12(6):544–50.
5. Barletta GM, Bunchman TE. Acute renal failure in children and infants. Curr Opin Crit Care. 2004;10:499–504.

6. Braun MC, Welch TR. Continuous venovenous hemodiafiltration in the treatment of acute hyperammonemia. Am J Nephrol. 1998;18(6):531–3.
7. Bunchman TE, Maxvold NJ, Kershaw DB, et al. Continuous venovenous hemodiafiltration in infants and children. Pediatr Nephrol. 1994;8:96–9.
8. Bunchman TE, McBryde KD, Mottes TE, et al. Pediatric acute renal failure: outcome by modality and disease. Pediatr Nephrol. 2001;16(12):1067–71.
9. Chen H, Yu RG, Yin NN, Zhou JA. Combination of extracorporeal membrane oxygenation and continuous renal replacement therapy in critically ill patients: a systemic review. Crit Care. 2014;18(6):675.
10. Flynn JT. Choice of dialysis modality for management of pediatric acute renal failure. Pediatr Nephrol. 2002;17:61–9.
11. Garist C, Favia Z, Ricci Z, Averadi M, Picardo S, Cruz DN. Acute kidney injury in the pediatric population. Contrib Nephrol. 2010;165:345–56.
12. Goldstein SL. Acute kidney injury in children: prevention, treatment, and rehabilitation. Contrib Nephrol. 2011:174:163–72.
13. Goldstein SL. Overview of pediatric renal replacement therapy in acute renal failure. Artif Organs. 2003;27(9):781–5.
14. Goldstein SL, Devarajan P. Acute kidney injury leads to pediatric patient mortality. Nat Rev Nephrol. 2010;6:393–4.
15. Goldstein SL, Currier H, Graf JM, et al. Outcome in children receiving continuous hemofiltration. Pediatrics. 2001;107(6):1309–12.
16. Hui-Stickle S, Brewer ED, Goldstein SL. Pediatric ARF epidemiology at a tertiary care center from 1999 to 2001. Am J Kidney Dis. 2005;45:96–101.
17. Kaufman J, Dhakal M, Patel B, Hamburger R. Community-acquired acute renal failure. Am J Kidney Dis. 1991;17(2):191–8.
18. Levy EM, Visconti CM, Horwitz RI. The effect of renal failure on mortality: a cohort analysis. JAMA. 1996:1489–94.
19. Markowitz GS, Perazella MA. Drug-induced renal failure: a focus on tubulointerstitial disease. Clin Chim Acta. 2005;351(1–2):31–47.
20. Maxvold NJ, Smoyer WE, Custer JR, Bunchman TE. Amino acid loss and nitrogen balance in critically ill children with acute renal failure: a comparison between CVVH and CVVHD therapies. Crit Care Med. 2000;28:1161–5.
21. Nash K, Hafeez A, Hou S. Hospital-acquired renal insufficiency. Am J Kidney Dis. 2002;39(5):930–6.
22. Nisula S, Kaukonen KM, Vaara ST, et al. Incidence, risk factors and 90-day mortality of patients with acute kidney injury in Finnish intensive care units: the FINNAKI study. Intensive Care Med. 2013;39:420–28.
23. Norman ME, Assadi F. A prospective study of acute renal failure in the newborn infant. Pediatrics. 1979;63:475–79.
24. Parekh RS, Bunchman TE. Dialysis support in the pediatric intensive care unit. Adv Ren Replace Ther. 1996;3:326–3.
25. Perazella MA. Drug-induced nephropathy: an update. Expert Opin Drug Saf. 2005;4(4):689–706.
26. Ronco C, Kellum JA, Mehta RL. Acute dialysis quality initiative (ADQI). Nephrol Dial Transplant. 2001;16(8):1555–8.

27. Ronco C, Tetta C, Mariano F, et al. Interpreting the mechanisms of continuous renal replacement therapy in sepsis: the peak concentration hypothesis. Artif Organs. 2003;27(9):792–801.
28. Ronco C, Ricci Z. Pediatric continuous renal replacement: 20 years later. Intensive Care Med. 2015;41(6):985–93.
29. Ronco C, Ricci Z, Goldstein SL. Revolution in the management of acute kidney injury in newborns. Am J Kidney Dis. 2015;May 7. Pil:S0272(15)00620-4. doi:10.1053/J.ajkd.2015.03.029 [Epub ahead of print].
30. Roy AK, Hoste EA, Clermont G, Kersten A, et al. RIFLE criteria for acute kidney injury is associated with hospital mortality in critically ill patients: a cohort analysis. Crit Care. 2006;10:R73.
31. Salahudeen AK, Doshi SM, Pawar T, Nowshad G, Lahoti A, Shah P. Incidence rate, clinical correlates, and outcomes of AKI in patients admitted to a comprehensive cancer center. Clin J Am Soc Nephrol. 2013;8:347–54.
32. Schetz M, Dasta J, Goldstein S, Golper T. Drug-induced acute kidney injury. Curr Opin Crit Care. 2005;11(6):555–65.
33. Tetta C, D'Intini V, Bellomo R, et al. Extracorporeal treatments in sepsis: are there new perspectives? Clin Nephrol. 2003;60(5):299–304.
34. Wan L. Bellomo R, Di Giantomasso D, Ronco C. The pathogenesis of septic acute renal failure. Curr Opin Crit Care. 2003;9(6):496–502.
35. Waikar SS, Liu KD, Chertow GM. Diagnosis, epidemiology and outcomes of acute kidney injury. Clin J Am Soc Nephrol. 2008;3:844–61.
36. Wang HE, Muntner P, Chertow GM, Warnock DG. Acute kidney injury and mortality in hospitalized patients. Am J Nephrol. 2012;35:349–55.
37. Warady B, Bunchman T. Dialysis therapy for children with acute renal failure: survey results. Pediatr Nephrol. 2000;15:11–3.
38. Williams DM, Sreedhar SS, Mickell JJ, et al. Acute kidney failure: a pediatric experience over 20 years. Arch Pediatr Adolesc Med. 2002;156:893–90.
39. Yang F. Zhang L, Wu H, Zou H, Du Y. Clinical analysis of cause, treatment and prognosis in acute kidney injury patients. PLoS. 2014;9(2):e85214. doi:10.1371/journal.pone.0085214.

Acute Kidney Injury

Definition

AKI (previously called acute renal failure) is characterized by abrupt onset of renal dysfunction manifesting as oliguria (urine output <0.5 mL/kg/h, for 6–12 h, a decrease in glomerular filtration rate (GFR) and the rise of serum creatinine) [3, 4, 14, 16, 26, 71]. The incidence of AKI in children appears to be increasing, and the etiology of AKI over the past decades has shifted from primary renal disease to multifactorial causes, particularly in hospitalized children [8, 13, 34, 42, 54, 70].

The history, physical examination, and laboratory studies, including urinalysis and radiographic studies, can establish the likely cause(s) of AKI. The prognosis of AKI is highly dependent on the underlying etiology of the AKI. Children who have suffered AKI from any cause are at risk for late development of kidney disease several years after the initial insult [20, 28, 29, 37, 71, 72].

Typically, in infants and small children, a minimal urine volume of approximately 1.0 mL/kg/h is required to excrete waste [16, 26, 43, 51]. Children with AKI due to hypoxic/ischemic insults, HUS, acute glomerulonephritis, and other causes are more likely to demonstrate oliguria or anuria (urine output less than 500 mL/24 h in older children or urine output less than 1 mL/kg/h in younger children and infants). Children with acute interstitial nephritis, nephrotoxic renal insults including aminoglycoside nephrotoxicity, and contrast nephropathy are more likely to have AKI with normal urine output. The morbidity and mortality rates of non-oliguric AKI are less than those of oliguric renal failure. While the precise incidence and causes of AKI in pediatric patients is unknown, recent studies suggest that the incidence of AKI in hospitalized children is increasing.

An important cause of AKI in hospitalized children is in the setting of post-cardiac surgery and in children undergoing stem cell transplantation. AKI in such children is frequently multifactorial, with ischemic/hypoxic injury and nephrotoxic insults being important contributors; the pathophysiology of hypoxic ischemic injury and nephrotoxic insults are described below [1, 14, 26, 28, 51, 68]. No epidemiology studies using an established definition of AKI have been conducted in pediatric patients. As described below, in pre-renal AKI the kidney is intrinsically normal, and renal function promptly returns to normal with restoration of adequate renal perfusion, while, in acute tubular necrosis (ATN), the kidney has sustained intrinsic injury, which requires repair and recovery before renal function returns to normal. Neonates with severe asphyxia had a higher incidence of AKI, while neonates with moderate asphyxia developed AKI less often.

In the urine output criteria, a urine output of less than 0.5 mL/kg/h for 8 h indicates the patient is at risk and should trigger the physician to start therapy [16].

This definition is, however, unreliable due to the lag time between the initiating injury and loss of kidney function, which may delay effective therapies that are limited to the early stage. Serum creatinine concentration does not increase until about 50 % of renal function is lost and also varies with age, muscle mass, medication, acid–base, and hydration status [8].

The RIFLE Criteria

In 2004, AKI Network and Kidney Disease Improving Global Outcome (KDIGO) introduced the risk, injury, failure, loss, and end-stage renal disease (RIFLE) classifications for the definition of AKI. RIFLE was modified for pediatric use (pRIFLE) (Table 1.1) [2, 52]. pRIFLE is a modification of the adult RIFLE

Table 1.1 Pediatric RIFLE criteria

	GFR criteria	Urine output criteria
Risk	eCCl decrease >25 %	<0.5 mL/kg/h × 8 h
Injury	eCCl decrease >50 %	<0.5 mL/kg/h × 16 h
Failure	eCCl decrease >75 %	0.3 mL/kg/h × 24 h or Anuria ×12 h
Loss	Complete loss of renal function >4 weeks	Complete loss of renal function >4 weeks
End-stage renal disease (ESRD)	ESRD >3 months	ESRD >3 months

References [2, 52]; *RIFLE* (R) risk, (I) injury, (F) failure,(L) loss, (E) end-stage renal disease, *GFR* glomerular filtration rate, *eCCl* estimated creatinine clearance, *ESRD* end-stage renal disease

classification and consists of three graded levels of injury (risk, injury, and failure) based upon the magnitude of change in estimated GFR (e.g., changes in serum creatinine) or urine output and two outcome measures, loss of kidney function and end-stage renal disease.

Small rises in serum creatinine levels of at least 0.3 mg/dL have been incorporated as the minimum requirements for the stage injury into the current definition of AKI.

The premise of the RIFLE criteria is to guide physicians on when to initiate therapy for the AKI patient. The first three letters R, I, and F allow the physician to assess patient AKI status and when to initiate therapy. Severity of AKI was graded from mild (RIFLE-R, "risk") to severe (RIFLE-F, "failure") based on changes in serum creatinine or estimated creatinine clearance and urine output. For example, a patient comes in with a serum creatinine of 1.0 mg/dL. A day later the patient's creatinine rises to 1.5 mg/dL. This patient should be placed in the risk category and therapy should be initiated [2, 52].

The last two letters, L and E, are considered outcome categories, and this basically indicates that if therapy at R, I, or F is not initiated, the mortality rate increases, or the patients will become dialysis dependent [2, 52]. Patients in the F category exhibit a higher mortality rate than those who were in the R and I category. This would indicate that R and I should trigger early initiation, which enhances survival rate. These efforts to standardize AKI definition are a substantial advance, although areas of uncertainty remain [2, 52].

Despite significant improvements in clinical care, the mortality and morbidity associated with AIK remains high (>50 %) and can lead to end-stage renal disease [20, 28, 29, 51, 70, 72]. The lag time between the initiating renal insult and loss of renal function as assessed based on serum creatinine may explain the high mortality and morbidity rates associated with the AKI. It is therefore desirable to have an alternative AKI biomarker less influenced by such errors yet capable of detecting minor degrees of renal impairment in the sick patients. Novel biomarkers may further refine the definition of AKI, but their use will need to produce tangible improvements in outcomes and cost effectiveness [5, 7, 8, 31].

Determination of Glomerular Filtration Rate

AKI alters both the pharmacokinetics and pharmacodynamics of the prescribed drugs. As the GFR decreases, the elimination of drugs that are primarily excreted by the kidneys also decreases proportionally. Thus, assessment of renal function is important and should include measurement of GFR.

The renal clearance of inulin is the most reliable method for determination of a true GFR, but its use is limited because of expense, lack of availability, and problems of collecting timed urine samples in infants and children. GFR estimation (eGFR) from the renal clearance of creatinine has been widely used in the pediatric population [57–62, 66]. Creatinine-based eGFR without urine collection has been used frequently in children. There are several ways to estimate GFR in children. One of the easiest and more practical one is Schwartz formula, which takes and uses the concept of height as a measure of muscle mass divided by serum creatinine [57, 58].

$$\text{eGFR}\left(\text{mL}/\text{min}/1.73\,\text{m}^2\right) = (K)(\text{height in cm}) / \text{serum creatinine}(\text{mg}/\text{dL})$$

The value of K is 0.45 for term infants throughout the first year of life, 0.55 for children up to17 years and adolescent girls, and 0.7 for adolescent boys [58–60].

In children, there is not a single formula recommended for all ages. Schwartz equation can be used to estimate GFR in children and adolescents but should be used with caution or avoided in premature infants in the first several months of life.

However, the use of Schwartz equation carries several limitations. First, with changing renal function, the serum creatinine concentration will no longer reflect the true eGFR. As a result, eGFR using Schwartz equation requires that renal function should be stable and that the serum creatinine measurement is constant. Second, the use of eGFR by Schwartz formula in patients with nutritional compromise as is common in children with cancer undergoing chemotherapy may overestimate the GFR values with subsequent overdosing of nephrotoxic agent. Similarly, in patients with CKD, falsely elevated creatinine clearance can occur due to the increase in external creatinine excretion [9]. The addition of cimetidine to inhibit tubular creatinine secretion permits accurate measurement of creatinine clearance in patients with CKD.

Recently, Schwartz et al. adapted the traditional Schwartz equation to children and adolescents but did not find different *k*-coefficients between children and adolescents [42]. De Souza and colleagues used linear mixed-effect models to reestimate the 2009 Schwartz *k*-coefficient in 360 consecutive French subjects aged 1–18 years [24]. They assessed the agreement between the estimated GFR obtained with the new Schwartz formula and the rate measured by inulin clearance. In De Souza, k was estimated at 0.325 in boys <13 years and all girls and at 0.365 in boys aged ≥ 13 years. The performance of this formula was higher than that of 2009 Schwartz formula in children <13 years. This was first supported by a statistically significant reduction of the overestimation of the measured GFR in both cohorts, by better 10

Table 1.2 Maximum AUC-based carboplatin dosage

Target AUC	Maximum carboplatin dose (mg)
6	900
5	750
4	600

Reference [67]

and 30 % accuracies, and by a better concordance correlation coefficient. These investigators concluded that the performance and simplicity of Schwartz formula are strong arguments for its routine use in children and adolescents. The specific coefficient for children aged <13 years further improves this performance.

Overestimation of GFR using creatinine-based equations have resulted in higher than intended carboplatin doses with a potential for increased toxicity. This concern for patients' safety led to the development of Calvert formula to determine the optimal carboplatin dosage [67]. Calvert formula is used to cap the maximum carboplatin dose based on target area under the curve (AUC). It is recommended that the maximum carboplatin dose should not exceed the target AUC (Table 1.2).

Calvert formula [67]: Total carboplatin dose (mg) = Target AUC (mg/mL/min) × creatinine clearance (mL/min) + 25.

Whereas the Schwartz formula is the widely used formula for the estimation of GFR in children, the Modification of Diet in Renal Disease (MDRD) and Cockcroft–Gault equations are the most popular estimate for adults but are inaccurate for patients less than 18 years old [25].

Radioisotopes such as ^{51}Cr-EDTA plasma disappearance are used in plasma disappearance GFR determinations; however, these are not ideal for use in children, especially for repeated studies [48]. The plasma disappearance of iohexol is a better alternative than ^{51}Cr-EDTA, because it is safe and not radioactive, easily measured, and freely excreted by glomerular filtration [48].

GFR estimating equations, based on serum concentrations of creatinine or cystatin C, are popular clinically and in research studies. To date, however, there is no dependable substitute for an accurately determined GFR, and iohexol plasma disappearance offers the best combination of safety, accuracy, and reproducible precision [60].

More recently, G. J. Schwartz and associates developed several new equations to estimate GFR in children using patient's height, serum creatinine, cystatin C, and blood urea nitrogen (BUN), of which the best equation, with the highest accuracy and correlation and the narrowest 95 % limits of agreement, was [61].

$$\text{eGFR} = 39.1 \times \left[\text{height}\left(\text{m}^2\right) / \text{SCr}\left(\text{mg}/\text{dL}\right)\right]^{0.516} \times \left[1.8 / \text{cystatin C}\left(\text{mg}/\text{L}\right)\right]^{0.294} \times \left[30 / \text{BUN}\left(\text{mg}/\text{dL}\right)\right]^{0.169} \times \left[1.099\ \text{male}\right] \times \left[\text{height}\left(\text{m}/1.4\right)\right]^{0.188}$$

These authors also described a simple bedside equation of 0.413 × height (cm)/serum creatinine (mg/dL), which provides a good approximation of eGFR in children and adolescents with CKD based on serum creatinine measurements referenced to the iohexol-based GFR determinations [61].

Urinary AKI Biomarkers

The incidence of both AKI and CKD is rising and reaching epidemic proportions [10]. In both situations, early intervention can significantly improve the dismal prognosis. Current standard assessments of renal function for pediatric patients use serum creatinine or formulas based on serum creatinine designed for longitudinal assessment of baseline renal function. It is accepted that the concentration of serum creatinine is an insensitive and delayed measure of decreased kidney function following AKI.

The accurate diagnosis of AKI is especially problematic in critically ill patients, in whom renal function is in an unsteady state, thus rendering such creatinine-based baseline assessment measures of renal function potentially inadequate.

Recently, a number of novel urinary AKI biomarkers including kidney injury molecule 1 (KIM-1), cystatin C (Cys-C), neutrophil gelatinase-associated lipocalin (NGAL), interleukin-18 (IL-18), and liver fatty acid-binding protein (L-FABP) have been identified and proved effective in predicting AKI prior to a change in serum creatinine levels [3–8, 13].

It is likely that they will be useful for timing the initial insult and assessing the duration and severity of disease (analogous to the cardiac panel for evaluating chest pain). Biomarkers may also serve to discern disease subtypes, identify etiologies, predict clinical outcomes, allow for risk stratification and prognostication, and monitor the response to interventions. The widespread availability of such information promises to revolutionize renal care in both children and adults and allow for the practice of personalized and predictive medicine at an unprecedented level.

Ischemic events, nephrotoxic drugs, and bacterial endotoxins are the frequent causes of AKI (about 90 %) [3, 4, 14, 16, 26, 28, 51, 68, 71, 72]. In these conditions, renal tubular injury is mediated through the release of pro-inflammatory cytokines and vasoactive substances leading to the necrosis of renal tubular epithelial cells [1]. ATN is followed by accumulation of biomarkers in the plasma and urine due to an increased synthesis in tubular cells (IL-18, KIM-1, NGAL) and/or impaired reabsorption in the proximal tubule (NGAL, cystatin C) [5, 7, 8, 31].

NGAL and IL-18 are pro-inflammatory cytokines that are produced and catabolized in the proximal tubule and have been reported as reliable markers of impaired proximal renal tubular dysfunction following ischemic and toxic injury, and after cardiac surgery, KIM-1 is known to mediate ischemic renal injury through activation of apoptosis in proximal renal tubular epithelial cells. Urinary KIM-1 appears to be more specific to ischemic or nephrotoxic injury and not significantly affected by prenatal azotemia, urinary tract infection, or CKD. Cys-C is a low-molecular-weight protein that is produced by all nucleated cells and freely filtered by glomerular filtration and then completely reabsorbed and catabolized by the healthy proximal tubular cells. Urine CYs-C levels increase when the proximal tubular cells are damaged. Sepsis and proteinuria may cause false-negative results [5, 7, 8, 31].

Of these biomarkers, NGAL, L-18, and KIM-1 have the highest potential for early diagnosis of AKI, and it is also recommended that a panel of biomarkers, rather than a single biomarker, will be needed to perform extremely well for mortality risk prediction after AKI [5, 7, 8, 31].

In children who underwent cardiac surgery, urinary NGAL concentration was highly predictive of subsequent clinical diagnosis of AKI (sensitivity 1.0, specificity 0.98), receiver operator characteristics (ROC) AUC=0.99 at 2 h after surgery. The AUC for urinary IL-18 ranges up to 0.9 for the early detection of AKI with low sensitivity but high specificity (0.85–0.94). Urinary KIM-1 level had an AUC of 0.80 for the early detection of ischemic urinary. KIM-1 concentrations were elevated to a much higher degree in patients with ischemic AKI than in patients with other forms of AKI with an AUC of 0.80.

Premature infants have higher levels of urinary AKI biomarkers compared with term infants because of the underdeveloped kidney function [3–5]. In recent studies, Askenazi et al. [2, 8] found that the baseline values of urine NGAL, KIM-1, and Cys-C but not IL-18 decreased with increasing gestational age. These authors found that the baseline urine NGAL, KIM-1, and Cys-C concentrations in premature infants (≤26 weeks' gestation) were 351 (ng/mL), 226 (pg/mL), and 911 (ng/mL), respectively. These values fell significantly to 85 (ng/mL), 143 (pg/mL), and 133 (ng/mL) for NGAL, KIM-1, and Cys-C, respectively, around 30 weeks of gestation. The mean urinary L-18 did not differ across gestational age categories and were 42 (pg/mL) for infants ≤26 weeks' gestation and 67 (pg/mL) ≥30 weeks' gestation, respectively. After the neonatal period, the median reference values for urine NGAL, KIM-1, and Cys-C are the following: 6.6 ng/mL, range 2.8–17; 410 pg/mL, range 226–703; and 20 ng/mL, range 0.5–200, respectively.

AKI Pathogenesis

Pre-renal azotemia and ischemic AKI are part of spectrum manifestations of renal hypoperfusion and can complicate any disease that reduces the "effective arterial blood volume" (e.g., cardiac failure, severe ischemia, hypovolemia) [1, 67]. Autoregulation of renal blood flow and GFR are overwhelmed at mean arterial blood pressure below 60–80 mmHg and AKI ensues. GFR may be impaired at lesser degrees of hypotension in neonates and those with preexisting renal diseases. Several drugs also perturb adaptive responses and can precipitate or aggravate pre-renal azotemia in subjects with renal hypoperfusion. These include nonsteroidal anti-inflammatory drugs (NSAIDs) and angiotensin-converting enzyme (ACE) inhibitors, which block biosynthesis of vasodilator prostaglandins and angiotensin II, respectively [38, 44, 55].

Patient-Related Risk Factors

Drug-induced renal disorders are more common in certain patients and in specific clinical situations. Infants and young children with extracellular volume depletion, sepsis, renal impairment, cardiovascular disease, diabetes, or prior exposure to radiocontrast agents are at risk of developing drug nephrotoxicity [72].

Drugs can cause AKI, intrarenal obstruction, interstitial nephritis, nephrotic syndrome, and acid–base and fluid–electrolyte disorders. Certain drugs can cause alteration in intraglomerular hemodynamics; inflammatory changes in renal tubular cells, leading to AKI; tubulointerstitial disease; and renal scarring. Drug-induced nephrotoxicity tends to occur more frequently in patients with intravascular volume depletion, diabetes, congestive heart failure, CKD, and sepsis [72]. Thus, early detection and treatment of drugs' adverse effects are important to prevent progression to end-stage renal disease. Table 1.3 provides list of the commonly used nephrotoxic drugs.

AKI Etiology

AKI has a long differential diagnosis. History can help to classify the pathophysiology of AKI as pre-renal, intrinsic renal, or post-renal failure, and it may suggest some specific etiologies.

Pre-renal Failure

Patients commonly present with symptoms related to hypovolemia, including thirst, decreased urine output, dizziness, and orthostatic hypotension. Ask about volume loss from vomiting, diarrhea, sweating, polyuria, or hemorrhage. Patients with advanced cardiac failure leading to depressed renal perfusion may present with orthopnea and paroxysmal nocturnal dyspnea.

Elders with vague mental status change are commonly found to have pre-renal or normotensive ischemic AKI. Insensible fluid losses can result in severe hypovolemia in patients with restricted fluid access and should be suspected in elderly patients and in comatose or sedated patients.

Pre-renal azotemia and ischemic AKI are part of spectrum manifestations of renal hypoperfusion and can complicate any disease that reduces the "effective arterial blood volume" (e.g., cardiac failure, severe systemic vasodilatation, hypovolemia) [1, 25]. Autoregulation of renal blood flow and GFR is overwhelmed at mean arterial blood pressure below 60–80 mmHg and AKI ensues. GFR may be impaired at lesser degrees of hypotension in neonates and those with preexisting renal diseases.

Pre-renal AKI represents the most common form of kidney injury and often leads to intrinsic AKI if it is not promptly corrected. Volume loss and decreased effective arterial blood volume can provoke this syndrome; the source of the loss may be

Table 1.3 The most commonly used nephrotoxic drugs[a]

Pre-renal azotemia	Acute tubular necrosis	Acute/chronic interstitial nephritis	Tubular obstruction	Hypersensitivity angiitis	Thrombotic microangiopathy
ACE inhibitors	ACE inhibitors	Acetaminophen	Acyclovir	Ampicillin	Clopidogrel
AT2-receptor antagonists	Acetaminophen	Acetazolamide	Ethylene glycol	Penicillin G	Cyclosporine
Cocaine	Aminoglycosides	Acetylsalicylic acid	Ganciclovir	Sulfonamides	Oral contraceptives
Cyclosporine	Amitriptyline	Acyclovir	Methotrexate		Quinine
Diuretics	Amphotericin B	Allopurinol	Probenecid		Mitomycin C
Estrogen	AT2-receptor antagonists	Ampicillin	Protease inhibitors		
Quinine	Cephalosporins	Cephalosporins	Quinolones		
Interleukins	Cisplatinum	Chlorpropamide	Sulfonamides		
Mitomycin C	Contrast media	Ciprofloxacin	Triamterene		
NSADIs	Cyclosporine	Cimetidine			
Tacrolimus	Dextran	Cisplatin			
	Diphenhydramine	Contrast media			
	Furosemide	Fenoprofen			
	Haloperidol	Furosemide			
	Mannitol	Indinavir			
	Methadone	Lansoprazole			
	NSAIDs	Lithium			
	Heavy metals	Methicillin			
	Pentamidine	Naproxen			
	Tacrolimus	NSAIDs			
	Tetracycline	Omeprazole			
		Oxacillin			
		Pantoprazole			
		Phenacetin			
		Phenindione			
		Phenytoin			
		Phenylbutazone			
		Ranitidine			
		Rifampicin			
		Sulfonamides			
		Thiazides			
		Vancomycin			

gastrointestinal, renal, or skin (e.g., burns) or from internal or external hemorrhage. Pre-renal AKI can also result from decreased renal perfusion in patients with heart failure or shock (e.g., sepsis, anaphylaxis).

Several classes of medications can induce pre-renal AKI in volume-depleted states, including ACE inhibitors, angiotensin receptor blockers (ARBs), aminoglycosides, amphotericin B, and radiologic contrast agents. Arteriolar vasoconstriction leading to pre-renal AKI can occur with the use of radiocontrast agents, NSAIDs, amphotericin, calcineurin inhibitors, norepinephrine, and other vasopressor agents.

The patient's age has significant implications for the differential diagnosis of AKI.

The most frequent cause of AKI in children and adolescents is under-perfusion of the normal kidney because of perinatal asphyxia. Various causes of hypovolemia and shock in the newborn may also result in AKI [1, 3, 4, 14].

To summarize, AKI can be caused by the following conditions:

Extracellular Volume Depletion

- Renal losses – diuretics, polyuria
- GI losses – vomiting, diarrhea
- Cutaneous losses – burns, Stevens–Johnson syndrome
- Hemorrhage

Decreased Cardiac Output

- Heart failure
- Pulmonary embolus
- Abdominal compartment syndrome – tense ascites

Systemic Vasodilation

- Sepsis
- Anaphylaxis
- Anesthetics
- Drug overdose

Afferent Arteriolar Vasoconstriction

- Hypercalcemia
- Drugs – NSAIDs, amphotericin B, calcineurin inhibitors, norepinephrine, radiocontrast agents
- Hepatorenal syndrome

Decrease Effective Arterial Blood Volume

- Hypovolemia
- Heart failure
- Liver failure
- Sepsis

Several measures of urinary parameters, including urine osmolality, urine sodium concentration, the fractional excretion of sodium, and the renal failure index, have all been proposed to be used to help differentiate pre-renal injury from hypoxic/ischemic AKI. Hypoxic/ischemic AKI is also called vasomotor nephropathy and/or

ATN, since there are early intense vascular constrictions followed by later tubular injury. Renal tubules are working appropriately in pre-renal injury and are able to conserve salt and water appropriately, whereas, in vasomotor nephropathy, the tubules have progressed to irreversible injury and are unable to conserve salt appropriately. During pre-renal injury, the tubules respond to decreased renal perfusion by appropriately conserving sodium and water such that the urine osmolality is greater than 400–500 mosmol/L, the urine sodium is less than 10–20 mEq/L, and the fractional excretion of sodium is less than 1 %.

Because the renal tubules in newborns and premature infants are relatively immature compared with those in older infants and children, the corresponding values suggestive of renal hypoperfusion are urine osmolality greater than 350 mosmol/L, urine sodium less than 20–30 mEq/L, and fractional excretion of sodium of less than 2.5 %. When the renal tubules have sustained injury, they cannot conserve sodium and water appropriately, so that the urine osmolality is less than 350 mosmol/L, the urine sodium is greater than 30–40 mEq/L, and the fractional excretion of sodium is greater than 2.0 %. The use of these values to differentiate pre-renal injury from ATN requires that the patient have normal tubular function initially. However, newborns with immature tubules and children with preexisting renal disease or salt-wasting renal adrenal disease, as well as other diseases, might have pre-renal injury with urinary indices suggestive of ATN but might, in reality, have pre-renal injury. Thus, it is essential that we consider the state of the function of the tubules before the potential onset that might precipitate vasomotor nephropathy/ATN, so that ascribing pre-renal injury to vasomotor nephropathy/ATN does not occur. In addition, the fractional excretion of sodium is often difficult to interpret in patients who have received diuretic therapy.

Intrinsic Renal Failure

Patients can be divided into those with glomerular etiologies and those with tubular etiologies of AKI. Nephritic syndrome of hematuria, edema, and hypertension indicates a glomerular etiology for AKI. Query about prior throat or skin infections. ATN should be suspected in any patient presenting after a period of hypotension secondary to cardiac arrest, hemorrhage, sepsis, drug overdose, or surgery.

A careful search for exposure to nephrotoxins should include a detailed list of all current medications and any recent radiologic examinations (e.g., exposure to radiologic contrast agents). Pigment-induced AKI should be suspected in patients with possible rhabdomyolysis (muscular pain, recent coma, seizure, intoxication, excessive exercise, limb ischemia) or hemolysis (recent blood transfusion). Allergic interstitial nephritis should be suspected with fevers, rash, arthralgia, and exposure to certain medications, including NSAIDs and antibiotics.

Structural injury in the kidney is the hallmark of intrinsic AKI; the most common form is ATN, either ischemic or cytotoxic. Glomerulonephritis can be a cause of AKI and usually falls into a class referred to as rapidly progressive glomerulonephritis (RPGN).

Ischemic AKI differs from pre-renal azotemia in that renal hypoperfusion has been severe enough to injure renal parenchymal cells, particularly tubule epithelium, and ARF does not resolve immediately after restoration of renal blood flow. Severe ischemia can induce bilateral renal cortical necrosis and irreversible renal failure. The distal portion of the proximal tubule and the medullary portion of the thick ascending limb of the loop of Henle are the nephron segments that are most vulnerable to ischemic injury. Both have high rates of active ATP-dependent solute transport and oxygen consumption. Furthermore, both are located in the outer medulla, an ischemic zone compared with other regions, even under normal conditions by virtue of the unique countercurrent arrangement of the medullary vasculature.

To summarize, vascular (large- and small-vessel) causes of intrinsic AKI include the following:

- Renal artery obstruction – thrombosis, emboli, dissection, vasculitis
- Renal vein obstruction – thrombosis
- Microangiopathy – TTP, HUS, disseminated intravascular coagulation (DIC)
- Malignant hypertension
- Transplant rejection

Glomerular causes include the following:

- Anti-glomerular basement membrane (GBM) disease – as part of Goodpasture syndrome or renal limited disease
- Anti-neutrophil cytoplasmic antibody-associated glomerulonephritis (ANCA-associated glomerulonephritis) – Wegener granulomatosis, Churg–Strauss syndrome, microscopic polyangiitis
- Immune complex glomerulonephritis – lupus, postinfectious glomerulonephritis, cryoglobulinemia, primary membranoproliferative glomerulonephritis

Tubular etiologies may include ischemia or cytotoxicity. Cytotoxic etiologies include the following:

- Heme pigment – rhabdomyolysis, intravascular hemolysis
- Crystals – tumor lysis syndrome, seizures, ethylene glycol poisoning, acyclovir, indinavir, methotrexate
- Drugs – aminoglycosides, lithium, amphotericin B, pentamidine, cisplatin, ifosfamide, radiocontrast agents

Interstitial causes include the following:

- Drugs – penicillins, cephalosporins, NSAIDs, proton-pump inhibitors, allopurinol, rifampin, indinavir, mesalamine, sulfonamides
- Infection – pyelonephritis, viral nephritides
- Systemic disease – lupus, lymphoma, leukemia, tubule-interstitial nephritis, uveitis

Post-renal Failure

Post-renal failure usually occurs in older men with prostatic obstruction and symptoms of urgency, frequency, and hesitancy. Patients may present with asymptomatic, high-grade urinary obstruction because of the chronicity of their symptoms. A history of prior gynecologic surgery or abdominal malignancy often can be helpful in providing clues to the level of obstruction.

Flank pain and hematuria should raise a concern about renal calculi or papillary necrosis as the source of urinary obstruction. Use of acyclovir, methotrexate, triamterene, indinavir, or sulfonamides implies the possibility that crystals of these medications have caused tubular obstruction.

To summarize, causes of post-renal AKI include the following:

- Ureteral obstruction – stone disease, tumor, fibrosis, ligation during pelvic surgery
- Bladder neck obstruction
- Urethral obstruction – strictures, tumor, phimosis
- Renal vein thrombosis

Diseases causing urinary obstruction from the level of the renal tubules to the urethra include the following:

- Tubular obstruction from crystals (e.g., uric acid, calcium oxalate, acyclovir, sulfonamide, methotrexate, myeloma light chains)
- Ureteral obstruction–ureteropelvic junction (UPJ) obstruction, ureterovesical junction (UVJ) obstruction, urolithiasis, or papillary necrosis
- Urethral obstruction–bladder neck obstruction, bladder stone, or neurogenic bladder

If the site of obstruction is unilateral, then a rise in the serum creatinine level may not be apparent, because of preserved function of the contralateral kidney. Nevertheless, even with unilateral obstruction, a significant loss of GFR occurs, and patients with partial obstruction may develop progressive loss of GFR if the obstruction is not relieved.

Bilateral obstruction is usually a result of prostate enlargement or tumors in men and urologic or gynecologic tumors in women. Patients who develop anuria typically have obstruction at the level of the bladder or downstream to it.

Etiology in Newborns and Infants

The most frequent cause of AKI in newborn infants is under-perfusion of the normal kidney because of perinatal asphyxia. Various causes of hypovolemia and shock in newborns may also result in AKI [1, 14, 54].

Pre-renal AKI

In newborns and infants, causes of pre-renal AKI include the following:

- Perinatal hemorrhage – twin–twin transfusion, complications of amniocentesis, abruptio placentae, and birth trauma.
- Neonatal hemorrhage – severe intraventricular hemorrhage and adrenal hemorrhage.

- Perinatal asphyxia and hyaline membrane disease (newborn respiratory distress syndrome) – both may result in preferential blood shunting away from the kidneys (e.g., pre-renal) to central circulation.

Intrinsic AKI

Hypoxic/ischemic AKI is characterized by early vasoconstriction followed by patchy tubular necrosis. Recent studies suggest that the vasculature of the kidney may play a role in acute injury and chronic injury as well, and the endothelial cell has been identified as a target of injury. Peritubular capillary blood flow has been shown to be abnormal during reperfusion, and there is also loss of normal endothelial cell function in association with distorted peritubular pericapillary morphology and function. The mechanism of cellular injury in hypoxic/ischemic AKI is not known, but alterations in endothelin or nitric oxide regulation of vascular tone, ATP depletion and alterations in the cytoskeleton, changes in heat shock proteins, initiation of the inflammatory response, and the generation of reactive oxygen and nitrogen molecules may each play a role in cell injury.

Nitric oxide is a vasodilator produced from endothelial nitric oxide synthase (eNOS), and nitric oxide helps regulate vascular tone and blood flow in the kidney. Recent studies suggest that loss of normal eNOS function occurs following ischemic/hypoxic injury which could precipitate vasoconstriction. In contrast, inducible nitric oxide synthase (iNOS) activity increases following hypoxic/ischemic injury, and iNOS can participate in the generation of reactive oxygen and nitrogen molecules. iNOS, with the generation of toxic nitric oxide metabolites including peroxynitrate, has been shown to mediate tubular injury in animal models of AKI. Endothelin (ET) peptides are potent vasoconstrictors that have also been shown to play a role in the pathogenesis of AKI in animal models. Endothelin receptor agonists for the A receptor have been shown to decrease AKI in animal models. Thus, alterations in the balance of vasoconstrictive and vasostimulatory stimuli are likely to be involved in the pathogenesis of hypoxic/ischemic AKI.

An initial response to hypoxic/ischemic AKI is ATP depletion, which leads to a number of detrimental biochemical and physiologic responses, including disruption of the normal cytoskeletal organization with loss of the apical brush border and loss of polarity with $Na^{+}K^{+}$ATPase localized to the apical as well as the basolateral membrane. This has been shown in several animal models of AKI, and it has also been shown in human renal allografts that loss of polarity with mislocation of $Na^{+}K^{+}$ATPase to the apical membrane contributes to kidney dysfunction in transplanted kidneys. Reactive oxygen molecules are also generated during reperfusion and can contribute to tissue injury. While tubular cells and endothelial cells are susceptible to injury by reactive oxygen molecules, studies have shown that endothelial cells are more sensitive to oxidant injury than tubular epithelial cells are. Other studies have shown an important role for heat shock protein in modifying the renal response to ischemic injury as well as playing a role in promoting recovery of the cytoskeleton following AKI.

In children with multiorgan failure, the systemic inflammatory response is thought to contribute to AKI as well as other organ dysfunction by the activation of the inflammatory response, including increased production of cytokines and reactive oxygen molecules, activation of polymorphonuclear leukocytes (PMNs), and increased expression of leukocyte adhesion molecules. Reactive oxygen molecules can be generated by several mechanisms including activated PMNs, which may cause injury by the generation of reactive oxygen molecules including superoxide anion, hydrogen peroxide, hydroxyl radical, hypochlorous acid, and peroxynitrite or by the release of proteolytic enzymes. Myeloperoxidase from activated PMNs converts hydrogen peroxide to hypochlorous acid, which may react with amine groups to form chloramines; each of these can oxidize proteins, DNA, and lipids, resulting in substantial tissue injury. Leukocyte endothelial cell adhesion molecules have been shown to be unregulated in ATN, and administration of anti-adhesion molecules can substantially decrease renal injury in animal models of ATN. As described below, several animal models have shown that interference with the inflammatory response may be the future therapy for hypoxic/ischemic AKI. Studies of humans with AKI have demonstrated an increased evidence of oxidation of proteins reflecting oxidant stress.

Causes of intrinsic AKI include the following:

- ATN – can occur in the setting of perinatal asphyxia; ATN also has been observed secondary to medications (e.g., aminoglycosides, NSAIDs) given to the mother perinatally.
- ACE inhibitors – can traverse the placenta, resulting in a hemodynamically mediated form of AKI.
- Acute glomerulonephritis – rare; most commonly the result of maternal–fetal transfer of antibodies against the neonate's glomeruli or transfer of chronic infections (syphilis, cytomegalovirus) associated with acute glomerulonephritis.

Post-renal AKI

Congenital malformations of the urinary collecting systems should be suspected in cases of post-renal AKI.

Etiology in Children

Pre-renal AKI

In children, gastroenteritis is the most common cause of hypovolemia and can result in pre-renal AKI. Congenital and acquired heart diseases are also important causes of decreased renal perfusion in this age group.

Intrinsic AKI

Intrinsic AKI may result from any of the following:

- Acute poststreptococcal glomerulonephritis – should be considered in any child who presents with hypertension, edema, hematuria, and renal failure
- HUS – often is cited as the most common cause of AKI in children

The most common form of HUS is associated with a diarrheal prodrome caused by *Escherichia coli* O157:H7. These children usually present with microangiopathic anemia, thrombocytopenia, colitis, mental status changes, and renal failure.

Drug-Induced AKI

Many medications including antibiotics, nonsteroidal anti-inflammatory agents, angiotensin-converting enzyme inhibitors, and radiocontrast agents can cause AKI as a result of direct tubular injury or alteration in intrarenal blood flow [17, 21, 22, 44–47, 49, 53, 54, 63, 64].

Nephrotoxin-induced AKI can complicate exposure to many structurally diverse poisons and to some endogenous compounds if present in the circulation at high concentrations (e.g., myoglobin, hemoglobin, and uric acid) [6, 14, 17, 20, 23, 38, 49, 51, 53, 55, 56, 63].

The kidney is especially vulnerable to nephrotoxic injury because of its rich blood supply and capacity to concentrate toxins within tubule epithelial cells and the interstitium via the actions of epithelial cell transports and renal countercurrent exchange [1]. As with ischemic AKI, nephrotoxins impair GFR by causing intrarenal vasoconstriction, direct injury to tubule epithelium, and tubule obstruction [23, 56]. Agents such as cyclosporine, radiocontrast compounds, myoglobinuria, and hemoglobinuria induce AKI by causing intrarenal vasoconstriction, whereas direct epithelial cell injury appears to be the primary event in AKI induced by many microbial agents (e.g., aminoglycosides, amphotericin B, cephalosporins, sulfonamide) and anticancer agents (e.g., cisplatin, ifosfamide) [17, 21, 32, 33, 38, 44, 46, 47, 49, 50, 53, 55, 63].

Several drugs also perturb adaptive responses and can precipitate or aggravate pre-renal azotemia in subjects with renal hypoperfusion [1]. These include NSAID and ACE inhibitors, which block biosynthesis of vasodilator prostaglandins and angiotensin II, respectively [6, 21, 22, 38, 39, 44, 45, 49, 50, 53, 55]. Because of slow excretion of drugs eliminated by the kidney during the neonatal period, toxic blood levels may easily be reached. The nephrotoxicity of aminoglycosides, amphotericin B, and radiocontrast agents is most likely due to the direct vasoconstriction and renal cytotoxicity. Aminoglycoside-induced vasoconstriction is most likely due to increased TXA2 synthesis, whereas oxygen free radicals seem to mediate contrast media-induced renal vasoconstriction [1]. Table 1.3 provides list of most frequently used nephrotoxic drugs.

Preventive measures require knowledge of mechanisms of drug-induced nephrotoxicity, understanding patients, and drug-related risk factors coupled with therapeutic intervention by correcting risk factors, assessing baseline renal function before initiation of therapy, adjusting the drug dosage, and avoiding use of nephrotoxic drug combinations.

Pathophysiologic mechanism of drug-induced nephrotoxicity is complex and often mediated through alteration of intraglomerular hemodynamics, impaired tubular secretion, inflammation, uric acid deposition, rhabdomyolysis, and thrombotic microangiopathy [17, 22, 23, 46, 47, 56]. Patients with underlying renal insufficiency, defined as GFR less than 60 mL/min/1.73 m^2, heart failure, sepsis, and intravascular depletion are particularly vulnerable to developing nephrotoxicity.

Aminoglycoside antibiotics, NSAIDs, contrast agents, and angiotensin-converting enzyme inhibitors (ACEI) are the most common causes of AKI in hospitalized patients [21, 38, 44, 45, 49, 53, 55, 63]. The risk of contrast-induced nephropathy is highest in diabetics and CKD diabetes [23, 56]. Drugs can also cause nephrotoxicity by altering intraglomerular hemodynamics and decreasing GFR [ACEI, angiotensin-converting enzyme blockers (ARBs), NSAID, cyclosporine, and tacrolimus] [1, 23, 56].

Drugs associated with AKI include aminoglycosides, amphotericin B, cisplatin, beta lactams, quinolones, rifampin, sulfonamides, vancomycin, acyclovir, and contrast agents [21, 38, 44, 45, 49, 53, 55, 63] (Table 1.3). These agents induce renal tubular cell injury by impairing mitochondrial function and interfering with tubular transport and increasing oxidative stress and free radicals [49, 53, 55]. Chronic use of acetaminophen, aspirin, diuretics, and lithium is associated with chronic interstitial nephritis leading to fibrosis and renal scarring [49, 63].

Certain drugs such as ampicillin, ciprofloxacin, sulfonamides, acyclovir, ganciclovir, methotrexate, and triamterene are associated with crystal nephropathy [32, 33, 46]. Crystal nephropathy may also result from the use of chemotherapy due to uric acid and calcium phosphate crystal deposition [23, 56].

Statins and alcohol may induce rhabdomyolysis because of a toxic effect on myocyte function [22]. Drugs most often associated with thrombotic microangiopathy include antiplatelet agents (e.g., cyclosporine, mitomycin C, and quinine) [47].

Children with cancer treated with cytotoxic drugs are frequently at risk of renal impairment. Anticancer therapy may cause glomerular and/or tubular injury, fluid–electrolyte disorders, renal Fanconi syndrome, and hemolytic uremic syndrome (Table 1.4) [32, 33, 46].

Mechanisms of anticancer drug-induced renal disorders generally include pre-renal hypoperfusion, intrinsic renal damage, damage to microvascular structure of the kidneys, hemolytic uremic syndrome, and intrarenal obstruction [23, 56].

AKI and electrolytes and acid–base imbalances are the most common adverse effects of anticancer treatments [32, 33, 46].

Mechanisms of anticancer drug-induced renal disorders generally include a varying degree of pre-renal hypoperfusion, intrinsic renal damage, renal tubular obstruction, and damage to microvascular structure of the kidneys [23, 56].

Patients with cancer are also frequently treated with nephrotoxic antibiotics including aminoglycosides, vancomycin, and amphotericin B. These patients may also undergo different radiologic studies with iodine contrast media and radiation therapy which themselves may cause nephrotoxicity [21].

Other risk factors potentiating renal dysfunction in cancer patients are extracellular volume depletion, preexisting renal impairment, sepsis, heart failure, and con-

Table 1.4 Nephrotoxicity associated with antineoplastic drugs[a]

Pre-renal azotemia	Glomerular disease (AKI)	Tubulointerstitial disease	Fanconi syndrome	Glomerular dysfunction	Hemolytic uremic syndrome
Cyclosporine	Carboplatin	Carboplatin	Azacitidine	Cisplatin	Cisplatin
Mitomycin C	Cisplatin	Cetuximab	Ifosfamide	Actinomycin D	Cyclosporine
Tacrolimus	Cyclosporine	Cisplatin	Streptozocin (nitrosourea)	IL-2	Gemcitabine
	Ifosfamide	Indinavir		Interferon alpha	Mitomycin C
	Interferon alpha	Ifosfamide		Melphalan	
	Methotrexate	Methotrexate		Methotrexate	
	Mitomycin C	Panitumumab		Nitrosoureas	
	Mithramycin			Pentostatin	
	Nitrosourea				
	Semustine (nitrosourea)				
	Tacrolimus				

[a]References [32, 33, 46]

comitant administration of nephrotoxic drugs including allopurinol and nonsteroidal anti-inflammatory agents [6, 17, 21, 51].

Nephrotoxicity induced by anticancer drugs can pose a significant challenge for both the nephrologist and oncologist. Therefore, assessing baseline renal function before initiation of therapy and during therapy, adjusting drug dosages, avoiding nephrotoxic drug combinations, and correcting risk factors are essential in cancer patients to avoid both acute life-threatening adverse effects and long-term toxicity that may cause permanent morbidity [11, 12, 15, 19, 36, 39, 63–65].

The cytotoxic drugs that most likely cause nephrotoxicity are cisplatin (CPL) and ifosfamide (IFO) that are used widely for cancer treatment in children. Renal toxicity is less frequent with other antineoplastic drugs but may occur from treatment with carboplatin methotrexate (MTX) and nitrosourea compounds (Table 1.4). General preventive measures should include the use of intravenous hydration, forced diuresis, and avoidance of known risk factors.

CPL can cause glomerular and tubular damage resulting in decreased GFR. The CPL nephrotoxicity is known to be a risk factor and may also be dose related [32, 33, 46]. Renal magnesium wasting, hypomagnesemia, hypokalemia, and hypocalcemia are the most common electrolyte disorders after CPL administration. Rising BUN and serum creatinine levels followed by AKI are generally noted after a bolus CPL administration $\geq$100 mg/m^2/day. Forced diuresis, combining hydration with furosemide, or mannitol administration has proved clinically beneficial to prevent kidney injury [11, 15, 36]. The carbonic anhydrase inhibitor acetazolamide has also been considered useful for prevention of contrast nephropathy and CPL nephrotoxicity [11]. Amifostine, sodium thiosulfate, and diethyldithiocarbamate also confer protection against CPL-induced renal dysfunction [33].

Carboplatin is a structural analogue of CPL. The combination of carboplatin and CPL is associated with more renal damage than the combination of CPL and IFO [32, 63].

Life-threatening carboplatin-associated toxicity may occur from errors in calculating GFR. To avoid this, it is recommended to dose carboplatin by the modified Calvert formula (Table 1.2). It takes under consideration creatinine clearance and the desired AUC [67].

IFO can also cause glomerular and tubular toxicity. Proximal tubular dysfunction is a prominent complication of ifosfamide therapy characterized by Fanconi syndrome and hypophosphatemic rickets [32, 64]. IFO dose greater than 100 g/m^2, age younger than 5 years, and combination therapy with CPL or carboplatin increase the risk of IFO-associated nephrotoxicity [32].

High-dose MTX can induce both glomerular and tubular dysfunctions leading to delayed elimination of the drug [46]. Precipitation of drug may occur in concentrated and acid urine resulting in renal tubular obstruction and AKI. Adequate hydration and urine alkalinization are the most important in preventing MTX-induced nephrotoxicity [11, 15, 36].

Monitoring the serum methotrexate level is necessary to prevent systemic toxicity including nephrotoxicity. Apart from vigorous hydration and alkalinization of urine, leucovorin should be administered in high-dose methotrexate therapy not only on the absolute drug serum level greater than 10^{-7} mol/L but also on the kinetics of these levels [11, 15, 36].

Prevention Strategies

Preventive strategies should target the safety of prescribing drug, monitoring their potential nephrotoxicity, correcting risk factors for nephrotoxicity.

Before initiation the drug therapy takes the following guidelines into consideration [11, 12, 15, 19, 36]:

1. Ensure adequate hydration and avoid the use of nephrotoxic drugs whenever possible.
2. Correct intravascular depletion to maintain renal perfusion before initiation of nephrotoxic agents.
3. Administer drug orally and use the lowest effective dose and shortest duration of therapy whenever possible.
4. Maintain drug levels within the recommended therapeutic range. Use less toxic analgesics with the lowest prostaglandin activity such as acetaminophen in patients with chronic pain and limit the duration of therapy.
5. Discontinue or reduce the dose of nephrotoxic drug with the first sign of toxicity. Monitor renal function and serum drug concentrations during drug therapy.
6. Use the lowest dose of low osmolar contrast agent in patients with preexisting renal insufficiency, heart failure, and diabetes. Ensure adequate hydration with normal saline or sodium bicarbonate infusion. Consider acetazolamide and monitor GFR 24–48 h postexposure.

Intravenous infusion of theophylline, given to severely asphyxiated neonates within the first hour of birth, was associated with improved fluid balance, creatinine clearance, and reduced serum creatinine levels and had no effects on neurological and respiratory complications. Adenosine is a potent vasoconstrictor that is released from the catabolism of ATP during ischemia; the potential mechanisms that theophylline could protect from AKI could be the blocking of the adenosine receptor. Other studies of asphyxiated neonates also demonstrated improved renal function and decreased excretion of beta-2 microglobulin in neonates given theophylline within 1 h of birth. However, the clinical significance of the improved renal function was not clear, and the incidence of persistent pulmonary hypertension was higher in the neonates who had received theophylline group. Additional studies are needed to determine the significance of these findings and the potential side effects of theophylline.

Diuretics and Dopamine Receptor Agonist

Diuretics and "renal-dose" dopamine are commonly used to prevent or limit AKI. There have been several clinical studies using mannitol, diuretics, and "renal-dose" dopamine for AKI. The stimulation of urine output eases management of AKI, but conversion of oliguric to non-oliguric AKI has not been shown to alter the course of renal failure. Furosemide may increase the urine flow rate to decrease intratubular obstruction and will inhibit Na-K-ATPase, which will limit oxygen consumption in already damaged tubules with a low oxygen supply. The use of "renal-dose" dopamine (0.5–3–5 μg/kg/min) to improve renal perfusion following an ischemic insult has become very common in intensive care units. While dopamine increases renal blood flow by promoting vasodilatation and may improve urine output by promoting natriuresis, there have been no definitive studies to demonstrate that low doses of dopamine are effective in decreasing the need for dialysis or improve survival times in patients with AKI. Fenoldopam is a potent, short-acting, selective, dopamine-1 receptor agonist that decreases vascular resistance while increasing renal blood flow. Fenoldopam has been used in a few children with AKI, including two children receiving therapy with a ventricular assist device as a bridge to cardiac transplantation; therapy with fenoldopam was thought to avoid the need for renal replacement therapy in one child.

The prognosis of AKI is highly dependent on the underlying etiology of the AKI. Children who have AKI as a component of multisystem failure have a much higher mortality rate than children with intrinsic renal disease such as HUS, RPGN, and AIN. Recovery from intrinsic renal disease is also highly dependent on the underlying etiology of the AKI. Children with nephrotoxic AKI and hypoxic/ischemic AKI usually recover normal renal function. In the past it has been thought that such patients are at a low risk for late complications, but several recent studies have demonstrated that CKD can evolve from AKI. Children who have suffered substantial loss of nephrons, as in HUS or RPGN, are at risk for late development of renal failure long after the initial insult has occurred. Several studies in animal models have documented that hyperfiltration of the remnant nephron may eventually lead to progressive glomerulosclerosis of the remaining nephrons. Thus, children who have had cortical necrosis during the neonatal period and whose renal function has recovered or children with an episode of severe Henoch–Schönlein purpura or HUS are clearly at risk for the late development of renal complications. Such children need lifelong monitoring of their renal function and blood pressure and lifelong urinalyses.

As described above, it has been thought that AKI due to hypoxic/ischemic and nephrotoxic insults were reversible, with a return of renal function to normal. However, recent studies have demonstrated that hypoxic/ischemic and nephrotoxic insults can lead to physiologic and morphologic alterations in the kidney that may lead to kidney disease at a later time. Thus, AKI from any cause can be a concern for later kidney disease. Importantly, AKI is likely to be especially deleterious when the kidney has not yet grown to adult size and/or before the full complement of nephrons have developed. Since nephrogenesis is not complete until approximately 34 weeks' gestation, AKI during this interval might lead to a decreased number of nephrons, and, indeed, studies have suggested that AKI during nephrogenesis results in decreased numbers of nephrons and subsequent glomerulomegaly. AKI in the full-term neonate is also associated with later kidney disease. In one study of six older children with a history of AKI not requiring dialysis in the neonatal period, only two were healthy, three had chronic renal failure, and one was on dialysis. Studies on older children have also shown that AKI leads to CKD in a higher percentage of children than was previously appreciated.

Table 1.5 Drug dosing in children with acute kidney injury[a]

Drug category	Protein binding (%)	$t_{(1/2)}$	Normal dose GFR 100 mL/min	Acute kidney injury GFR between 10 and 30 mL/min
Analgesic				
Acetaminophen	20–50	2–3	5 mg/kg iv q8h	Give normal dose q8h
Acetylsalicylic	>99	0.8	10 mg/kg q4–6h	Give normal dose q4–6h
Codeine	7	3	0.5–1 mg/kg q6h	75 % dose reduction q6h
Ibuprofen	90–99	1.8	5–10 mg/kg q6h	Give normal dose q6h
Ketorolac	>99	5	0.25–1 mg/kg q6h	Give normal dose q6h
Fentanyl	80–85	2.6	1–5 mcg/kg q6h	75 % dose reduction q6h
Meperidine	60–85	11	0.5–2 mg/kg iv infusion	75 % dose reduction iv infusion
Methadone	60–90	8–49	0.5 mg/kg iv q6h	Give normal dose q24h
Morphine	20–35	2.5	0.05–0.2 mg/kg iv q2–4h	75 % dose reduction q2–4h
Antibiotics				
Acyclovir	9–33	2–4	10 mg/kg iv q8h	Give normal dose q24h
Amikacin[b]	<20	0.2–0.7	20 mg/kg (max 1.5 g) iv q24h	Give 10 mg/kg iv and take trough level q24h and adjust the dose interval according to serum trough levels between 5 and 10 mg/L
Amphotericin	90	6–10	3–5 mg/kg iv q24h	Give normal dose iv q24h
Ampicillin	15–20	1–4	50 mg/kg (max 2 g) iv q8h	Give normal dose iv q8h
Azithromycin	10–15	6–8	5 mg/kg q12h	Give normal dose q12h
Aztreonam	50–60	2	80–120 mg/kg q8h	Give normal dose q8h
Benz penicillin	60	0.5–1	25–50 mg/kg iv q12h	Give normal dose iv q12h
Cefaclor	20–50	1	10–20 mg/kg iv q12h	Give normal dose iv q12h
Cefazolin	70–86	2	60–100 mg/kg q8h	Give normal dose q8h
Cefotaxime	40	1.5	50 mg/kg iv q8–12h	Give normal dose iv q8–12h
Ceftazidime	<10	1–2	25 mg/kg iv q8–12h	50 % dose reduction iv q24h
Ceftriaxone	85–95	8	80 mg/kg (max 4 g) iv q24h	Give normal dose iv q24h
Cefuroxime	33	1.5	25–50 mg/kg iv q8h	Give normal dose q12–24h
Cidofovir	<10	15–25	5 mg/kg iv q1–2 weeks	1 mg/kg iv q1–2 weeks
Ciprofloxacin	20–40	4–5	10 mg/kg iv q6h	50 % dose reduction q12h
Clindamycin	>90	2–3	5–10 mg/kg (max 1.2 g) iv q6h	Give normal dose iv q6h

(continued)

Table 1.5 (continued)

Drug category	Protein binding (%)	$t_{(1/2)}$	Normal dose GFR 100 mL/min	Acute kidney injury GFR between 10 and 30 mL/min
Co-amoxiclav	17–3	0.9	30 mg/kg (max 1.2 g) iv q8h	50 % dose reduction iv q12h
Co-trimoxazole (trimethoprim plus sulfamethoxazole)	60–66	5–17	40–60 mg/kg iv q12h	50 % dose reduction iv q12h
Erythromycin	70–95	2	12.5–25 mg/kg iv q6h	Give normal dose iv q12h
Flucloxacillin	95	2–3	25–100 mg/kg iv q8h	Give normal dose iv q8h
Fluconazole	12	15–20	6–12 mg/kg iv q48–72h	50 % dose reduction q48–72h
Ganciclovir	1–2	3–28	5 mg/kg iv q12h	50 % dose reduction q12h
Gentamicin[c]	1–30	1–3	7 mg/kg iv q24h	2–3 mg/kg iv q24h, take trough level after 4 and adjust the dose interval according to serum trough levels between 5 and 10 mg/dL
Imipenem	13–21	1–1.3	20–40 mg/kg (max 500 mg) iv q6h	50 % doe reduction iv q12h
Isoniazid	10–15	2.8	10–15 mg/kg q12–24h	Give normal dose q12–24h
Ketoconazole	85–99	8	3–6 mg/kg q24h	Give normal dose q24h
Levofloxacin	25–38	NA	5–10 mg/kg q24h	Give normal dose q24h
Meropenem	2	1.5–2	10–20 mg/kg iv q8h	50 % dose reduction iv q8h
Metronidazole	<20	6–12	7.5 mg/kg (max 500 mg) iv q8h	Give normal dose iv q8h
Nafcillin	90	1	15–50 mg/kg iv q12h	Give normal dose q12h
Flaxacillin	20–30	NA	15 mg/kg q12h	Give normal dose q12h
Piperacillin	20–30	0.7	200 mg/kg q4h	200 mg/kg q8h
Rifampicin	80	1–3.8	10 mg/kg iv q12h	Give normal dose iv q12h
Streptomycin	34	5–8	20–40 mg/kg iv q24h	7.5 mg/kg q24h
Ticarcillin	45–50	1.1	80 mg/kg iv (max 3.2 g) q8h	50 % dose reduction iv q8h
Vancomycin[b, c]	55	5.6	15 mg/kg iv q8h	10 mg/kg iv q12h, take trough level after 24 h, and adjust dose according to serum trough levels between 5 and 10 mg/L
Anticoagulants				
Heparin[d]	95	2	10–25 U/kg/h	Give normal dose
Warfarin	>90	50	0.5–8 mg q4h	Give normal dose q4h
Anticonvulsants				

(continued)

Table 1.5 (continued)

Drug category	Protein binding (%)	$t_{(1/2)}$	Normal dose GFR 100 mL/min	Acute kidney injury GFR between 10 and 30 mL/min
Carbamazepine	30	1.3	5–10 mg/kg q12h	75 % dose reduction q12h
Phenobarbital	30–50	80	3–7 mg/kg q24h	10 mg/kg q6–8h
Phenytoin	80–90	20	3–7 mg/kg q8h	Give normal dose q8h
Valproic acid	80–93	9–16	10–30 mg/kg q12h	Give normal dose q8h
Clobazam	83	18	10–30 mg q12h	Give normal dose
Clonazepam	85	30–40	0.01–0.1 mg/kg q8–12h	Give normal dose
Antihistamines				
Cimetidine	19	2	4–8 mg/kg q12h	50 % dose reduction q12h
Diphenhydramine	78	5–11	1 mg/kg q4–6h	Give normal dose q4–6h
Terbutaline	25	5.7	0.1–0.4 mg/kg/min iv infusion	Give normal dose
Antihypertensive agents				
Amlodipine	93	40	0.05–0.17 mg/kg q24h	Give normal dose q24h
Captopril	30	1.5	0.1–0.5 mg/kg q6–8h	75 % dose reduction q6–8h
Clonidine	20–40	8	2.5–5 mcg/kg q12h	Give normal dose q12h
Enalapril	<50	11	0.1 mg/kg q12h	75 % dose reduction q12h
Hydralazine	85–90	NA	0.05–0.2 mg/kg q8h	
Isradipine	95	1	0.5–0.2 mg/kg q8h	Give normal change q8h
Labetalol	50	NA	0.4–3 mg/h iv infusion	Give normal dose
Lisinopril	25	5–6	0.1 mg/kg q12–24h	50 % dose reduction q12–24h
Nifedipine	95	2.8	0.25–0.5 mg/kg q6–8h	Give normal change q6–8h
Prazosin	95	2.9	0.2–1 mg/kg q12h	Give normal change q12h
Propranolol	60–90	3.5	0.1–1 mg/kg q6h	Give normal dose q6h
Cardiovascular agents				
Amiodarone	96	NA	5–10 mg/kg q24h	Give normal dose q24h
Atenolol	<5	6	1–2 mg/kg q2h	Give normal dose q2h
Atropine	14–22	2–4	0.5–1 mg q5–30 min	Give normal dose
Digoxin	20–55	40	250 mcg q24h	62.5mcg q24h
Dobutamine	NA	2	2–20 mcg/kg/min iv infusion	Give normal dose
Dopamine	NA	5.5	2–20 mcg/kg/min iv infusion	Give normal dose
Epinephrine	NA	<0.1	0.01–1 mcg/kg/min iv infusion	Give normal dose
Milrinone	70	2.3	0.25–0.75 mcg/kg/min iv infusion	0.33 mcg/kg/min iv infusion

(continued)

Table 1.5 (continued)

Drug category	Protein binding (%)	$t_{(1/2)}$	Normal dose GFR 100 mL/min	Acute kidney injury GFR between 10 and 30 mL/min
Procainamide	15–20	3–4	20–80 mcg/kg/min iv infusion	Give normal dose
Verapamil	90	5	1–2 mg/kg q8h	Give normal dose q8h
Other				
Aminophylline	40	40	2 mg/kg q8h	Give normal dose q8h
Cytoxan[e]	13	7.5	Follow protocol	50–75 % dose reduction
Cyclosporine[b, c, e]	96	1	Follow protocol	No change
Dexamethasone	68	3	1–4 mg q6h	Give normal dose q6h
Hydrocortisone	70–90	1.7	5–10 mg/kg q6h	Give normal doseq6h
Insulin	98	0.3	0.5–10 U/h	Give normal dose
Mycophenolate	97	8–16	1 mg/m^2 q12h	Give normal dose q12h
Sirolimus	92	60	1 mg/m^2 q12h	Give normal dose q12h

[a]References [6, 11, 12, 15, 19, 39]; $t_{1/2}$ half time, *GFR* glomerular filtration rat, *iv* intravenous, *NA* not available
[b]Levels need to be checked daily
[d]Doses need to be adjusted according to APPT measured q12–24h
[e]According to protocol
[c]Subsequent doses should be based on the blood through level

Practical Considerations to Drug Dosing in AKI

Appropriate drug dosing in AKI is an important consideration to optimize therapeutic outcomes and to minimize drug toxicity. Underdiagnosed and untreated AKI may lead to CKD and end-stage renal disease [6, 11, 12, 15, 19, 39]. Guidelines whether or not dose adjustment is required for children with AKI are provided in Table 1.5.

Unlike cancer chemotherapy agents or antiepileptic drugs, most antibiotics have large therapeutic indices – that is, toxic doses far exceed therapeutic doses, and dose-limiting toxicities are rare. For example, vancomycin toxicity is frequently reported at concentrations in tenfold excess of the therapeutic concentration. Commonly encountered exceptions include aminoglycosides and amphotericin B, which concentrate in the renal cortex, causing AKI. Several azoles and macrolides are CYP3A4 inhibitors, and accumulation in renal failure may cause elevations in other drugs, especially immunosuppressants and antiarrhythmics, such as amiodarone, that are metabolized via CYP3A4. Beta-lactam antibiotics, especially carbapenems, have epileptogenic neurotoxicity that may be exacerbated by renal failure [33]. Because of these direct and indirect toxicities, practitioners have been keen to avoid overdose when prescribing antibiotics for patients with renal failure.

Dose adjustment in renal failure is usually based on the present level of renal function; however, estimation of renal function in acute renal failure is a challenging proposition that is becoming its own field of study. GFR estimates that are based on creatinine or urea levels, such as the MDRD estimating equation, are confounded by several factors. First, not all subjects generate wastes at the same rate. Second, measurements of serum levels always assess renal function "in arrears" as they reflect accumulation of the solute in the hours and days after the change in GFR occurred. Third, in AKI, the volume of distribution of these solutes is likely to also be changing rapidly, so that changes in plasma levels arise not just from changes in generation and in clearance but also changes in total body water. Several tools have been developed to quantify AKI in a repeatable fashion, and the most well known are the RIFLE and AKIN criteria. These tools were developed to standardize definitions and stages of AKI for research purposes, as previous studies of AKI were difficult to compare side by side due to widely varying definitions of AKI. These scoring systems are relatively blunt instruments with limited utility in bedside medical decision-making, although they are extremely helpful to the clinician's sense of risk stratification and anticipatory guidance to family and friends of the patient. In this background context of extraordinary difficulty in estimating renal function in the critically ill patient, rapid turnaround use of existing laboratory assays can be immensely useful. Four-hour creatinine clearance, for example, can give insight into a patient's renal function during the interval between administration of a loading dose and the first maintenance dose. These real-time assessments of actual creatinine clearance may prove helpful in estimating GFR when the patient's clinical condition is evolving.

The incidence of chronic renal disease and end-stage renal disease has nearly doubled over the last two decades across the globe. With annual mortality for patients on dialysis in the range of 20 % more, people die with treated uremia than with any cancer, except for lung cancer [36, 46, 63]. If current trends continue, the toll of ESRD will exceed that of lung cancer. The burden of disease is paralleled by the enormous cost for delivering end-stage renal disease care [10].

Medication dosing for children with AKI needs to be individualized based on pharmacokinetics and pharmacodynamics principles of the prescribed drugs whenever possible to optimize therapeutic outcome and to minimize toxicity. The pediatric RIFLE criteria should be prospectively utilized to identify patients at highest risk of developing AKI. AKI biomarkers such as serum creatinine and urine output along with volume status should be utilized to guide drug dosing when urinary biomarkers including kidney injury molecule 1, interleukin-18, or NGAL are not readily available [2, 4, 5]. Both the volume of distribution and half-life of several drugs are markedly increased in the presence of AKI and thus larger loading doses may need to be administered to achieve the target serum concentration. When possible, therapeutic drug monitoring should be utilized for those medications where serum drug concentrations can be obtained in a clinically relevant time frame. For those medications where therapeutic drug monitoring is available, close monitoring of drug blood level is highly recommended [12, 15, 36].

A practical approach to drug dosing in children with AKI begins with a complete history and physical examination. The history of previous drug allergy of toxicity and the use of the over-the-counter medications are important. Physical examination should include measurement of ideal body weight, estimating the extracellular volume, as the presence of edema or dehydration alters drug dosing [15].

The renal excretion of drugs depends on GFR and tubular reabsorption and secretion. The glomerular elimination of medications also depends on the molecular size and protein binding of the drugs. The renal elimination of drugs also is affected by the severity and etiology of renal disease.

Because of slow excretion of drugs eliminated by the kidney during the neonatal period, toxic blood levels may easily be reached. The nephrotoxicity of aminoglycosides, amphotericin B, and radiocontrast agents is most likely due to the direct vasoconstriction and renal cytotoxicity [1, 23, 56]. Aminoglycoside-induced vasoconstriction is most likely due to increased thromboxane A2 synthesis [23, 56].

If primarily kidneys excrete drugs, the renal elimination of drugs will be reduced and the drugs' plasma half-life will be prolonged in patients with AKI. As a result, drugs and their metabolites can accumulate in AKI patients and cause severe toxicity.

AKI patients typically have reduced oral intake and often require intravenous administration of drugs and fluid therapy. When adjusting drug doses for the AKI patient, drug doses should be adjusted based on the renal and non-renal clearance of the drug, the degree of renal impairment, and the potential nephrotoxicity of the concerned drug. The volume of distribution may be changed by AKI and critical illness. It is also necessary to know the degree of protein binding and the half-life of the concerned drug [50].

Because of the presence of a positive fluid balance in the early stages of AKI, the dosing regimen for many drugs, especially antimicrobial agents, should be initiated at normal or near-normal dosage regimens. In general, a loading dose that will achieve the target serum concentrations based on the expected volume of distribution should be given and no adjustments need to be made for residual renal function [12, 19].

References of Section Acute Kidney Injury

1. Abdelkader A, Ho J, Ow CP, Eppel GA, Rajapakse NW, Schlaich MP, et al. Renal oxygenation in acute renal ischemia-reperfusion injury. Am J Physiol Renal Physiol. 2014;306:F1026-38.
2. Akcan-Arikan A, Zappitelli M, Loftis LL, Washburn KK, Jefferson LS, Goldstein SL. Modified RIFLE criteria in critically ill children with acute kidney injury. Kidney Int. 2007;71:1028–35.
3. Andreoli SP. Acute renal failure. Curr Opin Pediatr. 2002;14:183–8.
4. Andreoli SP. Acute renal failure in the newborn. Semin Perinatol. 2004; 28(2):112–23.
5. Argyri I, Xanthos T, Varsami M, Aroni F, Papalois A, Dontas I, et al. The role of novel biomarkers in early diagnosis of acute kidney injury in newborns. Am J Perinatol. 2013;30:347–52.
6. Aronoff GR, Bennett WM, Berns J, Brier ME, Kasabaker N, Mueller BA, Pasko DA, Smoyer WA. Drug prescribing in renal failure: dosing guidelines for adults and children. 5th ed. Philadelphia: American College of Physicians; 2007.
7. Askenazi DJ, Koralkar R, Leviton EB, Goldstein SL, Devarajan P, Khandrika S, et al. Baseline values of candidate urine acute kidney injury (AKI) biomarkers vary by gestational age in premature infants. Pediatr Res. 2011;70:302–6.

8. Askenazi DJ, Montesanti A, Hunley H, Koralkar R, Pawar P, Shuaib F, et al. Urine biomarkers predict acute kidney injury and mortality in very low birth weight infants. J Pediatr. 2011;159:907–12.
9. Assadi F, John EG, Fornell L, Rosenthal I. Falsely elevated serum creatinine in ketoacidosis. J Pediatr.1985;107:562–4.
10. Assadi F. Strategies to reduce the incident of chronic kidney disease in children: time to change. J Nephrl.2012;26:41–7.
11. Assadi F. Acetazolamide for prevention of contrast-induced nephropathy. Pediatr Cardiol. 2006;27:237–42.
12. Assadi F. Medication dosing and renal insufficiency in a pediatric cardiac intensive unit. Pediatr Crdiol. 2008;29:1029–30.
13. Bagshaw SM. Epidemiology of renal recovery after acute renal failure. Curr Opin Crit Care. 2006;12(6):544–50.
14. Barletta GM, Bunchman TE. Acute renal failure in children and infants. Curr Opin Cri Care. 2004;10:499–504.
15. Barrett BJ, Parfrey PS. Clinical practice. Preventing nephropathy induced by contrast medium. N Engl J Med. 2006;354(4):379–86.
16. Bellomo R, Kellum JA, Ronco C. Defining acute renal failure: physiological principles. Intensive Care Med 2004; 30(1):33–7.
17. Briguori C, Airoldi F, D\drea D, et al. Renal insufficiency following contrast media administration trial (REMEDIAL): a randomized comparison of 3 preventive strategies. Circulation. 2007;115(10):1211–7.
18. Bunchman TE. Medication errors and patient complications with continuous renal replacement therapy. Pediatr Nephrol. 2006;21:842–45.
19. Bunchman TE, McBryde KD, Mottes TE, et al. Pediatric acute renal failure: outcome by modality and disease. Pediatr Nephrol. 2001;16(12): 1067–71.
20. Choudhury D, Ahmed Z. Drug-associated renal dysfunction and injury. Nat Clin Pract Nephrol. 2006;2(2):80–91.
21. Coco TJ, Klasner AE. Drug-induced rhabdomyolysis. Curr Opin Pediatr. 2004; 16(2):206–10.
22. Cummings BS, Schnellmann RG. Pathophysiology of nephrotoxic cell injury. In: Coffman TM, Falk RJ, Molitoris BA, editors. Schrier's diseases of the kidney. Philadelphia: Wolters Kluwer/Lippincott Williams & Wilkins; 2013. p. 868–900.
23. De Souza VC, Rabilloud M, Cochat P, Selistre L, Hadj-Aissa A, Kassai B, et al. Schwartz formula: is one k-coefficient adequate for all children? PLoS One. 2012;7(12):e5339.
24. Filler G, Foster J, Acker A, Lepage N, Akbari A, Ehrich JH. The Cockcroft-Gault formula should not be used in children. Kidney Int. 2005;67:2321–24.
25. Garist C, Favia Z, Ricci Z, Averadi M, Picardo S, Cruz DN. Acute kidney injury in the pediatric population. Contrib Nephrol. 2010;165:345–56.
26. Goldstein SL, Devarajan P. Acute kidney injury leads to pediatric patient mortality. Nat Rev Nephrol. 2010;6:393–4.
27. Goldstein SL, Currier H, Graf JM, et al. Outcome in children receiving continuous hemofiltration. Pediatrics. 2001;107(6):1309–12.

28. Han WK, Waiker SS, Johnson A, Betensky RA, Dent CL, Devarajan P, et al. Urinary biomarkers in the early detection of acute kidney injury. Kidney Int. 2008;73(7):863–9.
29. Hartmann JT, Fels LM, Franzke A, Knop S, Renn M, Maess B, et al. Comparative study of the acute nephrotoxicity from standard dose cisplatin +/– ifosfamide and high-dose chemotherapy with carboplatin and ifosfamide. Anticancer Res. 2000;20 3767–73.
30. Howell SB, Tactle R. Effect of sodium thiosulfate on cis-dichlorodiamineplatinum (II) toxicity and antitumor activity in L1210 leukemia. Cancer Threat Rep. 1980;64:611–16.
31. Hui-Stickle S, Brewer ED, Goldstein SL. Pediatric ARF epidemiology at a tertiary care center from 1999 to 2001. Am J Kidney Dis. 2005;45:96–101.
32. Kleber M, Cybulla M, Bauchmuller K, Ihorst G, Koch B, Engelhardt M. Monitoring of renal function in cancer patients: an ongoing challenge for clinical practice. Ann Oncol. 2007;18:950–8.
33. Levy EM, Visconti CM, Horwitz RI. The effect of renal failure on mortality: a cohort analysis. JAMA. 1996;275:1489–94.
34. Markowitz GS, Perazella MA. Drug-induced renal failure: a focus on tubulointerstitial disease. Clin Chim Acta. 2005;351(1–2):31–47.
35. Mattzke GR, Frye RF. Drug administrations in patients with renal insufficiency. Minimizing renal and extrarenal toxicity. Drug Saf. 1977;16:205–31.
36. Nisula S, Kaukonen KM, Vaara ST, et al. Incidence, risk factors and 90-day mortality of patients with acute kidney injury in Finnish intensive care units: the FINNAKI study. Intensive Care Med. 2013;39:420–28.
37. Norman ME, Assadi F. A prospective study of acute renal failure in the newborn infant. Pediatrics. 1979;63:475–79.
38. Perazella MA. Drug-induced nephropathy: an update. Expert Opin Drug Saf. 2005;4(4):689–706.
39. Perazella MA. Drug-induced nephropathy: an update. Expert Opin Drug Saf. 2005;4(4):689–706.
40. Perazella MA. Onco-nephrology: renal toxicities of chemotherapeutic agents. Clin J Am Soc Nephrol. 2012;7:1713–21.
41. Pisoni R, Ruggenenti P, Remuzzi G. Drug-induced thrombotic microangiopathy: incidence, prevention and management. Drug Saf. 2001;24(7): 491–501.
42. Rehling M, Moller ML, Thamdrup B, Lund JO, Trap-Jensen J. Simultaneous measurement of renal clearance and plasma clearance of ^{99m}Tc-labelled diethylenetriaminepenta-acetate, ^{51}Cr-labelled ethylenediaminetetra-acetate and inulin in man. Clin Sci. 1984;66:613–19.
43. Rennke, HG, Roos, PC, Wall, SG. Drug-induced interstitial nephritis with heavy glomerular proteinuria. N Engl J Med. 1980;302:691–2.
44. Roder, BL, Frimodt-Moller, N, Espersen, F, Rasmussen, SN. Dicloxacillin and flucloxacillin: pharmacokinetics, protein binding and serum bactericidal titers in healthy subjects after oral administration. Infection. 1995;23:107–12.

45. Ronco C, Bellomo R, Brendolan A, editors. Sepsis, kidney and multiple organ dysfunction (Contributions to Nephrology series, vol 144) and R.M. Lindsay (ed); U. Buoncristiani, R.S. Lockridge, A. Pierratos, G.O. Ting (co-eds): Daily and nocturnal hemodialysis (Contributions to Nephrology series, vol 145) Ronco et al. Karger, Basel; 2004, ISBN: 3-8055-7755-9.
46. Roy AK, Hoste EA, Clermont G, Kersten A, et al. RIFLE criteria for acute kidney injury is associated with hospital mortality in critically ill patients: a cohort analysis. Crit Care. 2006;10:R73.
47. Rossert J. Drug-induced acute interstitial nephritis. Kidney Int. 2001;60: 804–17.
48. Salahudeen AK, Doshi SM, Pawar T, Nowshad G, Lahoti A, Shah P. Incidence rate, clinical correlates, and outcomes of AKI in patients admitted to a comprehensive cancer center. Clin J Am Soc Nephrol. 2013;8:347–54.
48. Schetz M, Dasta J, Goldstein S, Golper T. Drug-induced acute kidney injury. Curr Opin Crit Care. 2005;11(6):555–65.
50. Schnellmann RG, Kelly KJ. Pathophysiology of nephrotoxic acute renal failure. In: Berl T, Bonventre JV, editors. Acute renal failure. Philadelphia, PA.: Blackwell Science; 1999. Schrier RW, editor. Atlas of diseases of the kidney, vol 1. http://www.kidneyatlas.org/book1/adk1_15.pdf. Accessed 8 Nov 2007.
51. Schwartz GJ, Feld LG, Langford DJ. A simple estimate of glomerular filtration rate in full-term infants during the first year of life. J Pediatr. 1984;104:849–54.
52. Schwartz GJ, Gauthier B. A simple estimate of glomerular filtration rate in adolescent boys. J Pediatr. 1985;106:522–26.
53. Schwartz GJ, Work DF. Measurement and estimation of GFR in children and adolescents. Clin J Am Soc Nephrol. 2009;4:1832–41.
54. Schwartz GJ, Furth S, Cole S, Warady B, Munoz A. Glomerular filtration rate via plasma iohexol disappearance: pilot study for chronic kidney disease in children. Kidney Int. 2006;69:2070–76.
55. Schwartz GJ, Munoz A, Schneider MF, Mak RH, Kaskel F, Warady BA, Furth SL. New equations to estimate GFR in children with CKD. J Am Soc Nephrol. 2009;20:629–37.
56. Schwartz GJ, Munoz A, Schneider MF, Mak RH, Kaskel F, et al. New equations to estimate GFR in children with CKD. J Am Soc Nephrol. 2009;20:629–37.
57. Skinner R, Parry A, Price L, Cole M, Craft AW, Pearson AD. Persistent nephrotoxicity during 10-year follow-up after cisplatin or carboplatin treatment in childhood: relevance of age and dose as risk factors. Eur J Cancer. 2009;45:3213–9.
58. Stöhr W, Paulides M, Bielack S, Jürgens H, Treuner J, Rossi R, et al. Ifosfamide-induced nephrotoxicity in 593 sarcoma patients: a report from the late effects surveillance system. Pediatr Blood Cancer. 2007;48:447–52.
59. Subach, RA, Marx, MA. Drug dosing in acute renal failure: the role of renal replacement therapy in altering drug pharmacokinetics. Adv Renal Replace Ther. 1998;5:141–7.
60. Vandrea Carla De Souza, Muriel Rabilloud, Pierre Cochat, Luciano Selistre, Aoumeur Hadj-Aissa, Behrouz Kassai, et al. Schwartz formula: is one k-coefficient adequate for all children? PLoS One. 2012;7(12):e5339.

61. van Warmerdam LJ, Rodenhuis S, ten Bokkel Huinink WW, Maes RA, Beijnen JH. The use of the Calvert formula to determine the optimal carboplatin dosage. J Cancer Res Clin Oncol. 1995;121(8):478–86.
62. Wan L, Bellomo R, Di Giantomasso D, Ronco C. The pathogenesis of septic acute renal failure. Curr Opin Crit Care. 2003;9(6):496–502.
63. Wang HE, Muntner P, Chertow GM, Warnock DG. Acute kidney injury and mortality in hospitalized patients. Am J Nephrol. 2012;35:349–55.
64. Williams DM, Sreedhar SS, Mickell JJ, et al. Acute kidney failure: a pediatric experience over 20 years. Arch Pediatr Adolesc Med. 2002;156:893–90.
65. Yang F, Zhang L, Wu H, Zou H, Du Y. Clinical analysis of cause, treatment and prognosis in acute kidney injury patients. PLoS. 2014;9(2):e85214. doi:10.1371/journal.pone.0085214.ecollection2014.

Chapter 2
Water and Solute Movements: Basic Physiology

Basic Concept of Solute Transport Mechanism

Water and solutes are transported through three different mechanisms: convection, diffusion, and ultrafiltration. The molecular size of the solute dictates which transport mechanism is required (Table 2.1). Molecular weights are measured in units called daltons. Urea, electrolytes, buffers, creatinine, glucose, and uric acid are a few examples of the "small"-molecular-size solutes (<350 Da). Vitamin B_{12} is a "middle"-molecule-size solute (1355 Da). Bilirubin, beta-2 microglobulin, myoglobin, and pro-inflammatory mediators of sepsis such as TNF-alpha, complement, and interleukin are all large-molecular-size solutes (5000–60,000 Da) (Table 2.1). Generally, the more a molecule weighs, the larger it is in size and the more resistant it is to transport [1–5].

Each CRRT modality provides at least one transport mechanism to move fluid and/or solutes out of or into the bloodstream. While ultrafiltration is used to transport fluid, there are three transport mechanisms to transport solutes: diffusion, convection, and adsorption. Understanding the principles of ultrafiltration, diffusion, convection, and adsorption helps to clarify which therapy or combination of therapies will best produce the desired outcome [1–3, 6–10].

Convection Transport Mechanism

Convection is defined as the movement of molecules across a semipermeable membrane due to a pressure gradient. The water pulls the molecule along with it as it follows through the membrane (solvent drag). In convection, plasma water moves along pressure gradients and will remove middle and large molecules [6, 8]. The pressure gradient in the extracellular circuit is increased by a positive pressure

F. Assadi, F.G. Sharbaf, *Pediatric Continuous Renal Replacement Therapy*,
DOI 10.1007/978-3-319-26202-4_2

Table 2.1 Solute molecular weights

Small molecular weights (daltons)	Middle molecular weights (daltons)	Large molecular weights (daltons)
Sodium (23)	Uric acid (168)	Inulin (5200)
Potassium (35)	Glucose (180)	Beta-2 microglobulin (11,800)
Urea (60)	Albumin/deferoxamine complex (700)	Inflammatory mediators (1200–40,000)
Creatinine (113)	Vitamin B_{12} (1355)	Albumin (55,000–60,000)

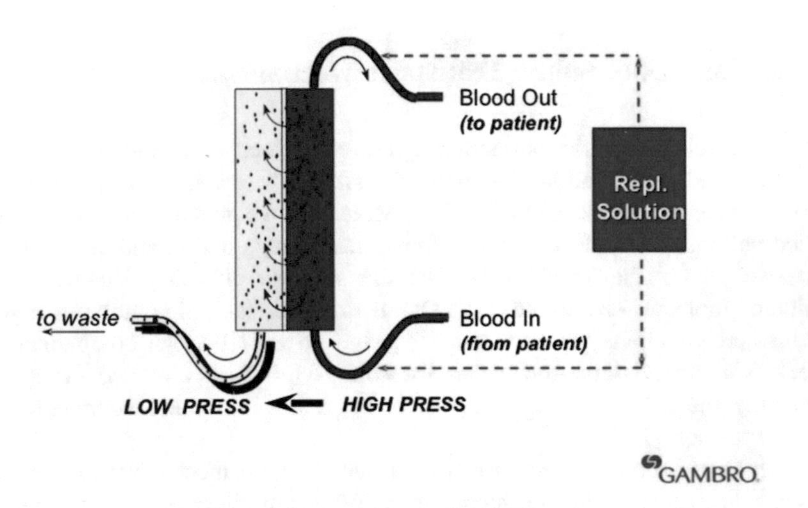

Fig. 2.1 Hemofiltration: convection transport mechanism (Gambro Training Manual, used with permission)

gradient (hydrostatic pressure) or oncotic pressure generated by non-permeable solutes (Fig. 2.1). Replacement fluid increases the amount of convective solute removal in CRRT. The effluent pump forces plasma water and solutes across the membrane in the filter. The fluid removed is referred to as "ultrafiltration." Ultrafiltrate is removed from the dialyzer and disposed of as effluent (Fig. 2.2). Increasing ultrafiltration rate will increase clearance by convection, and this requires more replacement solution. This transport mechanism is used in slow continuous ultrafiltration (SCUF), continuous veno-venous hemofiltration (CVVH), continuous veno-venous hemodialysis (CVVHD), and continuous veno-venous hemodiafiltration (CVVHDF) modalities [5, 11–13].

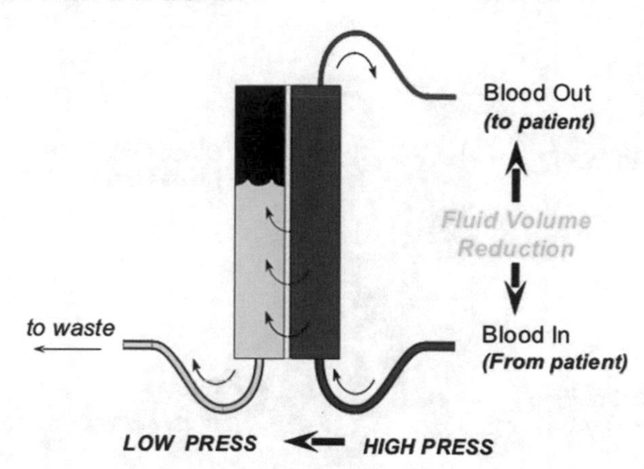

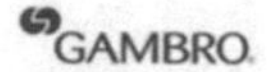

Fig. 2.2 Ultrafiltration: the movement of solutes from an area of higher pressure to an area of lower pressure (Gambro Training Manual, used with permission)

Diffusion Transport Mechanism

Diffusion is defined as the movement of solutes from an area of higher concentration to an area of lower concentration. In diffusion, the solvent moves by concentration gradient (Fig. 2.3). The solute gradually diffuses through the membrane from the area of high salt concentration to the area of low salt concentration (osmosis gradient) until it is evenly distributed. A uniform solution is created as seen in the cup on the left side of the membrane.

In the schematic, we can see how diffusion is created by dialysis therapy. Solutes travel from the area of high concentration on the blood side to the area of low concentration on the dialysate side (Fig. 2.3). The dialysate prescription is adjusted to preserve necessary solutes and remove unwanted solutes such as excess potassium or urea and creatinine. Note that dialysate flow is established countercurrent to the blood flow. This serves to increase effectiveness and maximize clearance [1, 2].

Plasma water and solutes are removed by diffusion and ultrafiltration and disposed of as effluent. Removal of small molecules is achieved by addition of dialysate to the fluid side of the filter. Dialysate is used to generate a concentration gradient across a semipermeable membrane. To increase clearance by diffusion, one should increase dialysate flow rate.

Dialysis therapy creates a concentration gradient across a semipermeable membrane (the filter) through which solutes diffuse selectively, based on particle size, as blood passes through the filter. Small solutes are removed efficiently by diffusion.

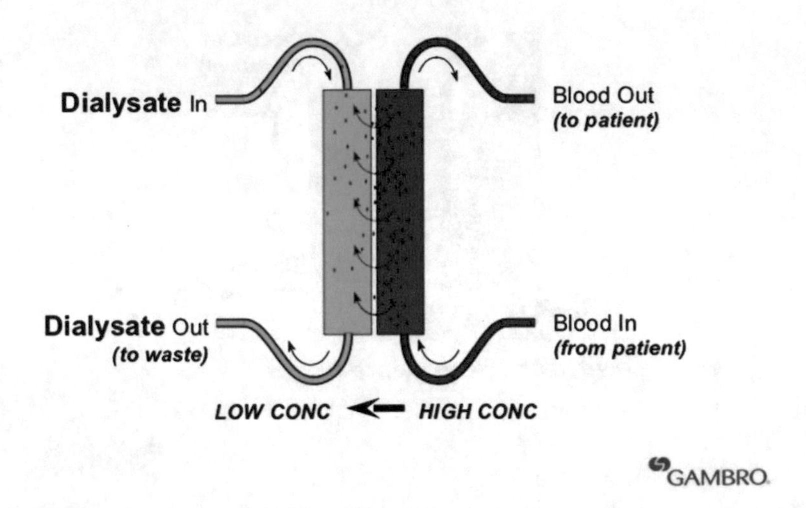

Fig. 2.3 Hemodialysis: diffusion transport (Gambro Training Manual, used with permission)

The reason why is that they are small enough to pass through the semipermeable membrane in response to a concentration gradient.

Diffusion is the solute transport mechanism used during dialysis. Small solutes, such as electrolytes, buffer, glucose, and metabolic waste products (urea or creatinine), are removed efficiently by diffusion and therefore by dialysis (Table 2.1).

CVVHD requires the use of blood, effluent, and dialysis pump. Replacement solution is not required. This transport mechanism is used in CVVHD and CVVHDF.

Hemofiltration (Convection) Versus Hemodialysis (Diffusion)

Convection is a process where solutes pass across a semipermeable membrane along with the solvent in response to a positive transmembrane pressure (TMP). Water is the solvent and the solutes small enough to pass through the pores of membrane are "dragged" along with the water as it is removed (Fig. 2.1). Removal of solutes, especially middle and large molecules, can be achieved by convection of relatively large volume of replacement fluid. This transport system is used in CVVHD and CVVHDF. Convection also drives adsorption of molecules, which we will discuss next (Table 2.1).

Convection is the main transport mechanism for middle and large molecules. Remember that inflammatory mediators fall into this size range but also myoglobin and bilirubin. Therefore, patients with elevated levels of myoglobin or bilirubin might be treated with a convective transport mechanism rather than diffusive in order to efficiently remove these solutes. The more fluid moved through a semipermeable membrane, the more solutes removed. From a practical point of view, convective transport is more effective for large-molecular-weight solutes such as protein and pro-inflammatory cytokines compared with diffusion transport system.

The difference in pressure between blood and replacement fluids creates a solvent drag for both small and large particle molecules across the membrane. The faster the replacement flow rates, the more solute is removed from blood. Ultrafiltrate is removed from the dialyzer and disposed of as effluent. CVVH requires blood, effluent, and replacement pumps. Dialysate is not required. Plasma and solutes are removed by convection and ultrafiltration.

Diffusion is solute transport across a semipermeable membrane. Molecules move from an area of higher concentration to an area of lower concentration. Diffusion is effective for small molecule clearance.

If we compare the efficiencies of diffusive and convective transport, we can say that diffusive transport, while excellent in the small-molecular-weight range, falls off rather rapidly in the middle- to large-molecular-weight range. Convective transport, on the other hand, offers clearance for middle to large molecules. These efficiencies become a major consideration when prescribing the optimal CRRT modality.

We have discussed the transport mechanism for removing fluid from blood. Now, we will review the transport mechanisms used to transport solutes. The molecular size of the solute dictates which transport mechanism is required. Generally, the more a molecule weighs, the larger it is in size and the more resistant it is to transport. This chart lists molecular weights for some of the common molecules that we are concerned with in CRRT. Molecular weights are measured in units called daltons.

Adsorption Transport Mechanism

Adsorption is the removal of solutes from the blood because they cling to the membrane. Think of an air filter. As the air passes through the filter, impurities cling to the filter itself and eventually the impurities will clog the filter and it will need to be changed. The same is true in blood purification. High levels of adsorption can cause the hemofilter to clog and become ineffective. The adsorption of solutes onto a membrane occurs as a result of the chemical properties of the membrane. These "adsorptive properties" may be influenced by electrical charge or the affinity of the membrane to "soak up" molecules similar to a sponge soaking up water. Surface adsorption allows for molecules too large to pass through the membrane to adhere on the surface of the membrane. Molecules that adhere to the membrane will be removed from circulation. Bulk adsorption describes the adsorption of molecules that are small enough to pass through the membrane but actually is retained in the structure of the membrane. Overall, adsorption causes limited removal of some solute across the membrane and high levels of adsorption may cause the membrane to clog. This mechanism is used in SCUF, CVVH, CVVHD, and CVVHDF. Studies show that TNF-alpha is removed mainly by adsorption versus convection or diffusion.

The primary goal of CRRT is to regain renal function and discharge the patient from the hospital as soon as possible. Continuous maintenance of fluid, electrolyte, and acid–base balance is of primary consideration. It has been well established that when treating patients in AKI or those requiring renal support, allowing them to become hypotensive during therapy can lengthen the healing process, prolong the onset (resolution) of AKI, and even send the patients into end-stage renal disease. Therefore, preventing complications that are damaging to the kidneys, such as hypotension, is another important goal.

References

1. Bellomo R. Choosing a therapeutic modality: hemofiltration vs. hemodialysis vs. hemodiafiltration. Semin Dial. 1996;9:88–92.
2. Braun MC, Welch TR. Continuous venovenous hemodiafiltration in the treatment of acute hyperammonemia. Am J Nephrol. 1998;18(6):531–3.
3. Brunet S, Leblanc M, Geadah D, et al. Diffusive and convective solute clearances during continuous renal replacement therapy at various dialysate and ultrafiltration flow rates. Am J Kidney Dis. 1999;34:486–92.
4. Parakininkas D, Greenbaum LA. Comparison of solute clearance in three modes of continuous renal replacement therapy. Pediatr Crit Care Med. 2004;5(3):269–74.
5. Siegler MH, Teehan BP. Solute transport in continuous hemodialysis: a new treatment for acute renal failure. Kidney Int. 1987;32:562–71.
6. Bunchman TE, Maxvold NJ, Kershaw DB, et al. Continuous venovenous hemodiafiltration in infants and children. Am J Kidney Dis. 1995;25:17. Infants and Children, Pediatr Nephrol 1994;8:96–9.
7. Davies SP, Reaveley DA, Brown EA, Kox WJ. Amino acid clearance and daily losses in patients with acute renal failure treated by continuous arteriovenous hemodialysis. Crit Care Med. 1991;19(12):1510–5.
8. Goldstein SL. Continuous renal replacement therapy: mechanism of clearance, fluid removal, indications and outcomes. Curr Opin Pediatr. 2011;23:181–5.
9. Hmiel SP, Martin RA, Landt M, et al. Amino acid clearance during acute metabolic decompensation in maple syrup urine disease treated with continuous venovenous hemodialysis with filtration. Pediatr Crit Care Med. 2004;5(3):278–81.
10. Meyer TW, Walther JL, Pagtalunan ME, et al. The clearance of protein bound solutes by hemofiltration and hemodiafiltration. Kidney Int. 2005;68(2):867–77.
11. Golper TA. Continuous arteriovenous hemofiltration in acute renal failure. Am J Kidney Dis. 1985;6(6):373–86.
12. Jiang HL, Xue WJ, Li DQ, et al. Pre- vs. post-dilution CVVH. Blood Purif. 2005;23(4):338.
13. Ronco C, Kellum JA, Mehta RL. Acute dialysis quality initiative (ADQI). Nephrol Dial Transplant. 2001;16(8):1555–8.

Chapter 3
Continuous Renal Replacement Therapy (CRRT)

Principle of Continuous Renal Replacement Therapy

Dialytic intervention for infants and children with acute kidney injury (AKI) can take many forms [1–12]. Whether patients are treated by intermittent hemodialysis, peritoneal dialysis, or continuous renal replacement therapy (CRRT) depends on specific patient characteristics [13]. Modality choice is also determined by a variety of factors, including provider preference, available institutional resources, dialytic goals, and the specific advantages or disadvantages of each modality [14–25]. Our approach to AKI has benefited from the derivation and generally accepted defining criteria put forth by the Acute Dialysis Quality Initiative (ADQI) group [18]. These are known as the risk, injury, failure, loss, and end-stage renal disease (RIFLE) criteria. A modified pediatrics' RIFLE (pRIFLE) criteria have recently been validated. Common defining criteria will allow comparative investigation into therapeutic benefits of different dialytic interventions [2].

While this is an extremely important development in our approach to AKI, several fundamental questions remain. Of these, arguably, the most important are "When and what type of dialytic modality should be used in the treatment of pediatric AKI?"

The choice of an appropriate modality for AKI depends on the clinical status of the patient as well as the dialytic indication. Clinically, several important patient conditions require attention. Initial patient assessment should focus on whether multiple organ systems are involved and to what extent. A patient with AKI solely will predictably have a better potential outcome than those with multisystem failure. If AKI is the only morbidity associated with the patient, then it is important that quantification of urine output (if present) be acknowledged. This will help determine the patient's ability to handle fluid and solute load. Classically defined indicators for RRT initiation in the setting of AKI are extrapolations of those we have commonly used for end-stage renal disease (ESRD) and include metabolic/electrolyte imbalance, uremia with bleeding and/or encephalopathy, hypervolemia with pulmonary edema/respiratory failure, intoxications, inborn errors of metabolism, and nutritional support.

F. Assadi, F.G. Sharbaf, *Pediatric Continuous Renal Replacement Therapy*,
DOI 10.1007/978-3-319-26202-4_3

While these may be recognized indicators, to date there has been no adequate definition of what "timing of initiation" means. The decision to initiate RRT may be affected by strongly held physician beliefs (in terms of indications), patient characteristics (including age/size, illness acuity, and comorbidities), and organizational characteristics (including resource availability, type of institution, type of ICU, type of provider, and perceived cost of therapy). All these factors will ultimately determine the appropriateness and availability of modality choice.

Specific indications for RRT typically include the need for ultrafiltration (i.e., fluid removal), either for symptomatic volume overload or to make space for nutrition, medications, and blood product support and/or solute removal (i.e., urea, potassium), either for uremia or for removal of a dialyzable toxin [5, 24, 26–41]. In addition to these clinical variables, the use of specific modalities in terms of need for nutritional support to aid in patient recovery from AKI or its underlying cause must be considered. The rapid removal of solute (urea) and correction of electrolyte abnormalities (particularly elevated levels of potassium) are of extreme importance in the setting of AKI. While peritoneal dialysis (PD), intermittent hemodialysis (IHD), and CRRT can rapidly correct hyperkalemia and uremia, IHD and CRRT provide greater clearance of higher-molecular-weight solutes than PD [13, 14, 40, 42–44]. The rapidity of solute generation and its particular urgency for removal, as in tumor lysis syndrome, inborn error of metabolism, hyperammonemia, symptomatic hyperkalemia, or ingestion of dialyzable toxins, require IHD or CRRT rather than PD, whereas mild uremia can be treated with any of the modalities. Urgent fluid removal required in patients with pulmonary edema and difficulty in ventilating may only be achieved by IHD or CRRT. Mild volume overload can be treated with any modality. For example, a hemodynamically unstable patient with overwhelming sepsis, fluid overload, respiratory compromise, pressor requirements, and renal involvement may necessitate initiation of CRRT for close fluid status control, whereas a postoperative cardiac patient with minimal fluid overload and hemodynamic instability may be better served by PD. The physical characteristics of the type of solute to be removed (e.g., molecular size, percentage of protein binding) may determine the need for IHD versus PD versus CRRT (CVVH vs. CVVHD). The metabolic status of the patient may also reflect the type of dialytic solution required (Table 3.1). [5, 23, 24, 26–41, 47].

The physical condition of a patient in terms of underlying disease process, size, previous surgical procedures, and overall stability will often dictate choice of modality. Contraindications to PD may include diaphragmatic hernia, recent intra-abdominal surgery, intra-abdominal sepsis, lack of an adequate peritoneal surface, or intra-abdominal malignancy. Also, in AKI secondary to HUS, gut involvement may be severe enough to preclude PD, as may necrotizing enterocolitis in a neonate. Severe hypotension may prohibit the use of IHD. A patient's size may prevent successful vascular access or even temporary PD. Indeed, in our smallest neonates, vascular access may not be achievable with double-lumen catheters in the neck or groin, and single lumen 5 Fr. catheters may need to be placed in the umbilical vessels. In the same neonatal patient, even temporary PD may be impossible when automated machinery is used, due to tubing "dead space." Such considerations must be taken

Table 3.1 Mechanisms of solute removal: intermittent hemodialysis versus continuous renal replacement therapy[a]

Solutes	Intermittent hemodialysis	CRRT
Small solutes (MW < 300)	Diffusion[b]	Diffusion[c] (CVVHD) Convection (CVVH)
Middle molecules (MW 500–5000)	Diffusion Convection	Convection Diffusion
Large molecules (MW 5000–50,000)	Convection Adsorption	Convection Adsorption
Large proteins (MW > 50,000)	Convection	Convection

[a]References [27, 32, 45, 46]
[b]Determinants: flow rates, membrane thickness
[c]Determinants: effluent dialysate flow rate

into account in determining the feasibility of dialysis delivery in our smallest patients. The presence of a coagulopathy may impact on performance of IHD or CRRT or the ability to establish vascular access for either modality.

CRRT is a mode of renal replacement therapy that is used for hemodynamic instable, fluid overload, and septic patients complicated by AKI in the critical care/intensive care unit setting [16, 22, 27, 30, 36, 45, 48–55]. CRRT provides a slow, gentle treatment of AKI and fluid removal much like the native kidney (ultrafiltration up to 120 mL/h) and is generally well tolerated by critically ill, hemodynamically unstable patients. The CRRT is intended to substitute for impaired renal function over an extended period of time and applied for 24 h a day. It provides slower solute clearance per unit time as compared with intermittent hemodialysis therapies, but over 24 h may even exceed clearances with intermittent hemodialysis.

Peritoneal or intermittent hemodialysis is not suitable for patients suffering from sepsis because it cannot remove the inflammatory mediators (large-molecular-weight particles). In addition, critically ill neonates and infants with recent abdominal surgery and compromised cardiopulmonary function often are unable to tolerate peritoneal therapy. Likewise, hemodynamically unstable children may not tolerate rapid ultrafiltration with conventional hemodialysis therapy [3, 10–12, 22, 26, 28, 40, 43, 45, 52–54, 56–64].

CRRT differs considerably from intermittent hemodialysis, relying heavily upon continuous ultrafiltration of plasma water. It has the potential for removal of large quantities of larger-molecular-weight drugs, such as glycopeptide antibiotics, from plasma [13]. Moreover, control of anemia, acid–base balance, and fluid volume can be achieved easily and continuously maintained with CRRT. In addition, CRRT removes inflammatory mediators of sepsis such as TNF-alpha, interleukin, and complement [60]. CRRT is also used to allow other supportive measures, such as nutritional support. Feeding patients in critical care may require large amounts of fluid. CRRT offers a fluid balance mechanism, ultrafiltration, to assist with balancing fluid and to remove metabolic waste products [24, 33–35, 65–68].

CRRT is usually performed through a double-lumen venous hemodialysis catheter situated in a large vein (usually an internal jugular), an extracorporeal circuit, a hemofilter, a blood pump, and an effluent pump to establish a steady blood flow into the circuit either as hemofiltration (CVVH), hemodialysis (CVVHD), or a combination of the two: hemodiafiltration (CVVHDF) [1, 4, 5, 19, 29, 53, 57, 69–73].

CRRT technique may differ significantly according to the mechanism of solute transport, the type of membrane, the presence or absence of dialysate solution, and the type of vascular access. CVVH and CVVHD are the two most commonly used hemofiltration techniques for treatment of neonatal AKI [29, 74].

CVVH uses a predominantly hydrostatic pressure gradient (convection) to pump solute across a filter membrane to achieve clearance.

CVVHD, on the other hand, uses diffusion across a membrane to effect clearance of solute. This is achieved by generating a continuous concentration gradient using countercurrent flow of plasma and dialysate fluid, between which equilibration occurs. However, the filtration flow rates in CVVHD are relatively low because its effectiveness in drug clearance is mainly achieved through diffusion. As a result, drugs with a higher molecular weight are removed more slowly and show a lower clearance than drugs with smaller molecular weight. CVVHDF uses a combination of the connective (ultrafiltration) and diffusion (dialysis) techniques to remove solutes.

The impact of CRRT on drug removal is variable depending on the various techniques that are used in the management of AKI, the ultrafiltrate and dialysate flow rates, the filter, and the patients' residual renal and non-renal drug clearance.

In general, drugs that are predominately removed by the normal kidneys require a dose reduction in patients with AKI. If CRRT is initiated, some of the drugs may be eliminated by CRRT. The extent of drug removal determines whether supplemental dosing is necessary during CRRT to avoid the drug underdosing (see sections "Drug Removal During CRRT: Basic Principles," "Drug Dosing During CRRT," and "Factors Influencing the Clearance of Drugs During CRRT").

Advantages of Continuous Renal Replacement Therapy

CRRT has several theoretical advantages over intermittent blood purification techniques, including better hemodynamic tolerability, more efficient solute clearance, better control of intravascular volume, and better clearance of middle and large-molecular-weight substances.

Hypotension is one of the most common complications associated with intermittent hemodialysis, occurring in approximately 20–30 % of all treatments. Some of the causes are dialysis specific, such as excessive or rapid volume removal, changes in plasma osmolality, and autonomic dysfunction. In critically ill patients who may be hemodynamically unstable, it would be desirable to minimize this complication, as it may lead to further organ ischemia and injury. Several prospective and retrospective studies have demonstrated better hemodynamic stability associated with CRRT [13, 20, 42, 43, 53, 75]; however, this observation has not been validated in a randomized controlled trial.

Another advantage of CRRT is the improved efficiency of solute removal. Although the clearance rate of small solutes is slower per unit time with CRRT (17 mL/min vs. more than 160 mL/min with conventional hemodialysis), CRRT is continuously administered; therefore, urea clearance is more efficient after 48 h than with alternate-day intermittent hemodialysis. Clark et al. developed a computer model based on 20 critically ill patients to compare solute clearance in intermittent and continuous renal replacement therapies and found that for a 50 kg male, an average of four dialysis sessions/week would be required to achieve equivalent uremic control [17]. In patients with a weight greater than 90 kg, equivalent uremic control could not be achieved with intermittent therapies even if daily dialysis was prescribed.

Fluid management is often a difficult issue in ICU, where nutritional requirements (TPN) and the use of IV medications necessitate the administration of large amounts of fluid to critically ill patients. The inability to severely restrict fluid intake in ICU patients results in excessive volume overload, which may compromise tissue perfusion and has been associated with adverse outcomes [33, 34, 49]. Attempts to restrict fluid in this setting may additionally compromise adequate nutrition. The capacity to adjust fluid balance on an hourly basis, even in hemodynamically unstable patients, is largely responsible for the growing popularity of CRRT.

CRRT may also have an immunomodulatory effect. The rationale for the use of CRRT for the treatment of sepsis arises from the observed association between sepsis severity mortality rate and serum concentrations of various cytokines including TNF, IL1, IL6, and IL8. Most of these middle-molecular-weight molecules are water-soluble and are theoretically removable by hemofiltration-based plasma water purification [40, 60, 67]. At the present time the immunomodulatory effects of CRRT remain theoretical and have not been shown to affect outcome in human studies [65].

Despite its apparent advantages over intermittent therapies, superiority of CRRT with respect to mortality or recovery of renal function has not been demonstrated. In the largest randomized controlled trial to date ($n=166$), intermittent hemodialysis was associated with significantly lower in-hospital (48 vs. 65 %) and ICU mortality (42 vs. 60 %). However, patients with hypotension were excluded from participating in the study, and there was a significant difference in severity scores between the treatment arms despite randomization [13, 23, 45, 76]. Two recently published meta-analyses compared intermittent with continuous renal replacement therapies in unselected critically ill patients [23, 76]. Both concluded that there was no difference in terms of renal recovery. However, while Kellum concluded that there was improved survival with CRRT [23], Tonelli found no survival benefit with either modality [76]. Moreover, the sample size required showing a 20 % mortality difference between intermittent hemodialysis and CRRT would be in excess of 1200 patients.

There are also significant cost implications associated with modality choice for treatment of ARF in the ICU setting. A study comparing CRRT to alternate-day IHD showed CRRT to be significantly more expensive, primarily because of the cost of CRRT fluid. Cost differences also depend on whether these procedures are performed by critical care nurses or by renal unit nurses and whether interunit charges are applied. Further studies are needed to define the subset of patients with ARF who benefit from this therapy.

Indications for CRRT

The precise decision of CRRT initiation is usually a matter of clinical judgment and depends upon patient hemodynamic stability, the availability of vascular access, and supporting nursing staff and technical resources [5, 77–80]. Hemofiltration is usually indicated in children with anuric AKI complicated by edema, electrolytes abnormalities, catabolic patients with increased nutritional needs, patients with septic shock, inborn error of metabolism, diuretic unresponsive edema, poisoning, and hepatic coma.

Absolute indications for dialysis include symptoms or signs of uremia (e.g., changes in mental status, pericardial rub or effusion, uremic platelet dysfunction) and management of volume overload, hyperkalemia >6 mEq/L with ECG changes, or metabolic acidosis (pH < 7.15) that is refractory to medical therapy [27, 32, 45, 46].

A. Renal Causes [27]

1. AKI with septicemia, fluid overload, cardiovascular instability, and pulmonary edema
2. AKI with electrolytes and acid–base imbalance
3. Oliguric AKI with high fluid requirements (nutrition, blood products)

B. Non-renal Causes [32, 45, 46]

1. Inborn errors of metabolism (hyperammonemia, lactic acidosis)
2. Systemic inflammatory response syndrome
3. Acute cardiopulmonary failure with fluid overload
4. Intoxication
5. Hepatic or drug-induced coma
6. Severe burns
7. Post-organ transplants

CRRT is indicated in the pediatric population for hypervolemic anuric AKI, electrolyte abnormalities, catabolic patients with increased nutritional needs, patients with sepsis, poisoning, inborn errors of metabolism, diuretic unresponsive hypervolemia, and hepatic or drug-induced coma. Intoxicants amenable to hemofiltration are vancomycin, methanol, procainamide, thallium, lithium, methotrexate, and carbamazepine.

Severe sepsis and septic shock are the primary causes of multiple organ dysfunction syndrome including AKI. Variety of water-soluble mediators with pro- and anti-inflammatory activities such as INF, IL-6, IL-8, and IL-10 play a major role in the pathogenesis of septic shock leading to the activation of the complement cascade and coagulation pathways. Early CVVH/CVVHD interventions utilizing higher ultrafiltration rate greater than 35 mL/kg/h coupled with adsorption to a membrane with increasing pore size to enhance middle molecule have shown to improve removal of water-soluble sepsis mediators.

Additionally, hemofiltration (HF) in conjunction with other therapies such as extracorporeal membranous oxygenation (ECMO), patients with cardiomyopathy on a left-ventricular assist device (LVAD), and the newer hepatic support therapies has also proven to be quite useful [6, 16, 17, 48].

Practical Considerations for Pediatric CRRT

Peritoneal or intermittent hemodialysis dialysis is not suitable for patients suffering from sepsis because it cannot remove the inflammatory mediators (large-molecular-weight particles) [13, 15]. Furthermore, critically ill neonates and infants with recent abdominal surgery and compromised cardiopulmonary function often are unable to tolerate peritoneal therapy. Likewise, hemodynamically unstable children may not tolerate rapid ultrafiltration with conventional hemodialysis therapy.

CRRT provides a slow, gentle treatment of AKI and fluid removal much like the native kidney (ultrafiltration up to 120 mL/h) [1–3, 14, 20, 35, 52–55, 69, 71, 73, 81–83]. Moreover, control of azotemia, acid–base balance, and fluid volume can be achieved easily and continuously maintained with CRRT. CRRT provides a slow, gentle treatment of AKI and fluid removal much like the native kidney and is generally well tolerated by critically ill, hemodynamically unstable patients. In addition, CRRT removes inflammatory mediators of sepsis such as TNF-alpha, interleukin and complement. CRRT is also used to allow other supportive measures, such as nutritional support. Feeding patients in critical care may require large amounts of fluid. CRRT offers a fluid balance mechanism, ultrafiltration, to assist with balancing fluid and to remove metabolic waste products [6, 7, 9, 25, 40, 42–44, 47, 59, 61, 63, 75, 78, 79, 84–87].

Timing of CRRT

There is no commonly accepted definition for the timing of initiating renal replacement therapy in AKI, although several observational and retrospective analyses have suggested improved survival with earlier initiation of renal support [70, 88].

It has been suggested that patient outcome can be improved by early or more intensive dialysis to keep the BUN under 80–100 mg/dL (29–36 mmol/L). However, because the BUN may reflect many factors other than the timing of initiation, no absolute value for BUN or creatinine should be used to determine when to initiate dialysis.

Only one randomized controlled trial has looked at the effect of timing of initiation of renal replacement therapy on outcome [56]. Bouman et al. randomized 106 critically ill patients with ARF to early versus late initiation of dialysis. Early initiation was started within 12 h of patients meeting the following criteria: low urine output (<30 cc/h) × 6 h refractory to optimization of hemodynamics and diuretics and creatinine clearance of <20 mL/min. The late initiation group was started on dialysis when the classic indications for dialysis were met (volume overload, hyperkalemia, urea greater than 40 mmol/L). There was no significant difference between the groups in terms of ICU or hospital mortality and no difference with respect to recovery of renal function. The results of this study must be interpreted with some caution, however, as the study was underpowered to detect a clinically significant difference and the mortality rate in all treatment groups was very low.

The dialysis working group consensus statement on renal replacement therapy makes no recommendations on the timing of initiation of renal replacement therapy beyond those defined by the conventional criteria that apply to chronic renal failure [18].

Kinetic Modeling of Solute Clearance

At the present time, a urea kinetic model (UKM)-based calculation of plasma solute clearance is the most common method measurement of dialysis dosage with both intermittent and continuous forms of dialysis, although it is not entirely clear that the calculated clearance values can be directly compared. This calculation is called *Kt/V*, where *K* is clearance, *t* is duration of dialysis, and *V* is the volume of distribution of urea.

$$K = \text{Removal rate}\left(\text{solute out} - \text{solute in}\right) / \text{concentration}$$

$$K \text{ for most CRRT circuits} = V \times \text{CU}_F / C_B,$$

$$\text{CU}_F / C_B = \text{Sieving Coefficient and for most solute is} \sim 1.0.$$

CVVH sieving coefficient for sodium and potassium are 0.99, chloride 1.05, bicarbonate 1.12, BUN 1.05, creatinine 1.02, glucose 1.04, calcium 0.64, magnesium 0.90, phosphate 1.04, albumin 0.01, and total protein 0.02.

$$V = \text{Effluent rate}\left(\text{Dialysis rate} + \text{ultrafiltration rate}\right)$$

The limitation of this method rests in the observation that critically ill patients with ARF are frequently catabolic and have highly variable fluid volumes; both conditions violate several of the assumptions implicit in urea kinetic modeling.

CRRT Dosing Recommendation

Similarly, there is no consensus as to what the minimal dialysis dose should be in patients with AKI. It seems reasonable to suggest a minimum *Kt/V* of 1.2 should be delivered at least three times a week in patients with AKI. However, several recent studies support the belief that more intensive dialysis may be beneficial in this patient group. A randomized dose-intensity study of CVVH in 425 critically ill patients demonstrated a significant decrease in patient mortality when ultrafiltration rates of 35 mL/kg/h were used as compared with 20 mL/kg/h [7, 74, 86, 89]. A randomized trial of intermittent hemodialysis comparing daily with alternate-day dialysis showed a reduction in mortality from 46 to 28 % ($p<0.05$). Unfortunately the delivered dialysis dose in the alternative day group as measured by weekly *Kt*/*V* was less than 3.6, the minimally acceptable dose in chronic dialysis patients, thus the issue of minimal adequate dose remains unresolved.

CRRT Modality Choice

CRRT solute clearance is dependent on the molecular size of the solute, the pore size of the semipermeable membrane, and the type of CRRT modality. The higher the ultrafiltration rate, the greater is the solute clearance.

CRRT can be performed with ultrafiltration (SCUF), hemofiltration (CVVH), or hemodialysis (CVVHD) or a combination of both techniques (CVVHDF). Of these the CVVH and CVVHD are often used in children requiring CRRT [1, 3, 7, 8, 23, 25, 42, 56, 63, 69, 73, 75–77, 87, 90, 91].

Arteriovenous modes of CRRT using the patient's own cardiac output to drive blood flow through the dialysis circuit are no longer used due to the development of external circuit pump and the high access complications rate [1, 3, 55].

Small-molecular-weight substances, such as urea, is cleared equally by both diffusive and connective modes (CVVH, CVVHD, CVVHDF), but for large-molecular-weight substances such as proteins, vancomycin, or cytokine clearance, the convection mode (CVVH) is superior over the diffusive mode of therapy [5, 26, 28, 39, 40, 47, 60, 74, 92]. In septic and highly catabolic patients, there is an advantage of convective over diffusive clearance [39, 40, 74]. There is always a greater risk of underdosing medications and sieving nutrition from patients with the convection than diffusion mode of therapy.

Slow Continuous Ultrafiltration

Slow continuous ultrafiltration (SCUF) is the simplest CRRT modality that aims for excess fluid volume removal without administration of a replacement solution. Mechanism of water transport in SCUF is ultrafiltration. Primary indication for SCUF is management of fluid overload without metabolic imbalance. The amount of fluid and its composition in the effluent bag are the same as the amount of fluid removed from the patient.

In SCUF blood enters the extracorporeal circuit through an access line, passes through the hemofilter, and returns to the patient circulation via the return line [4, 5,

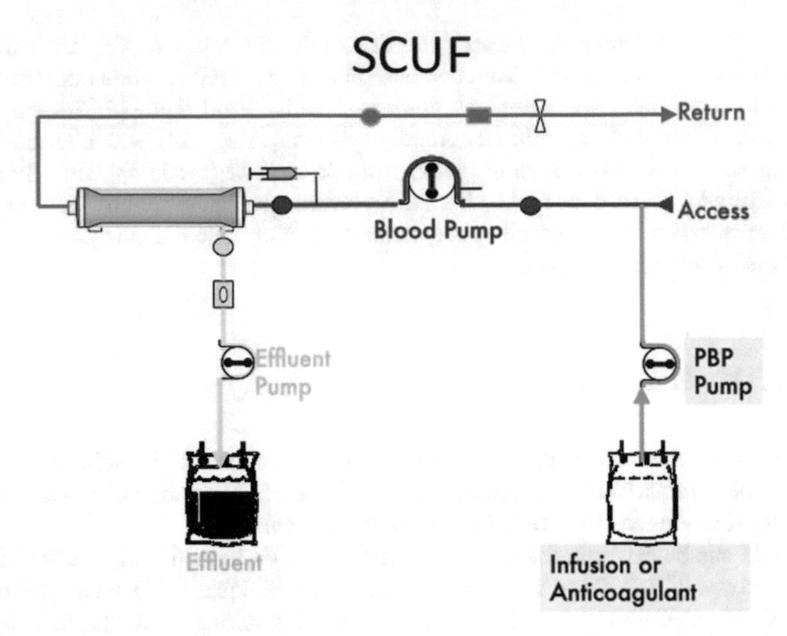

Fig. 3.1 Slow continuous ultrafiltration (SCUF) (Gambro Training Manual, used with permission)

39, 74]. Here is the schematic for SCUF. Notice the blood pump, effluent pump, and the PBP which are accessible (Fig. 3.1).

As the blood passes through the filter, ultrafiltration takes place and effluent collects in the effluent bag. Effluent is any fluid that exits the hemofilter and is delivered to a waste bag [17]. Pumps control blood flow and fluid removal rates. The maximum patient fluid removal rate is 200 mL/h.

Small molecules easily pass through a membrane driven by diffusion and convection. Middle- and large-size molecules are cleared primarily by convection. Semipermeable membrane removes solutes with a molecular weight of up to 50,000 Da. Plasma proteins or substances highly protein-bound will not be cleared.

The sole objective of SCUF therapy is to provide fluid balance in the patient by removing plasma water, up to 2000 mL/h, through ultrafiltration across a semipermeable membrane. SCUF requires a blood and an effluent pump. SCUF is useful for safe and large fluid removal in patients with congestive heart failure who is fluid overloaded and does not respond to diuretics but does not require solute balance. Safe fluid removal up to 2 L/h can be achieved.

The patient fluid removal rate may be set to balance the effects of infusions to the patient, such as parenteral nutrition or drug administration, or to correct a fluid overload condition. Blood flow rate may be set between 18 and 180 mL/min. The effluent dose is recommended at 35 mL/kg/h. This type of ultrafiltration utilizes no replacement or countercurrent replacement solution (dialysate), but only removes fluid. The patient fluid removal rate is the net amount that the system removes from the patient each hour. SCUF is usually performed at ultrafiltration rates below 8 mL/min. Although it is very rare to have a patient who can tolerate high fluid removal rates, the SCUF system can remove up to 2 L of fluid per hour from the patient.

This therapy might be used for a patient who is simply fluid overloaded but does not require solute balance, for example, a patient with congestive heart failure admitted with fluid overload. They do not respond well to their diuretics. If their kidneys cannot excrete excess fluid, SCUF can do the job.

Continuous Veno-venous Hemofiltration (CVVH)

CVVH is a highly effective method of solute removal and is indicated for uremia, severe metabolic acidosis, or electrolyte imbalance with or without fluid overload. CVVH is particularly efficient at removing small and large molecules (e.g., B12, TNF) via convection utilizing a pre- and/or post-filter replacement solution at about 35 mL/kg/h. Solutes can be removed in large quantities while easily maintaining a net zero or even a positive fluid balance in the patient. The amount of fluid in the effluent bag is equal to the amount of fluid removed from the patient plus the volume of replacement fluids administered. No dialysis solution is used [1, 5, 28, 39, 49, 56, 72, 74, 93].

CVVH adds use of pumped replacement fluids, either pre- or post-filter, to enhance middle molecule clearance by convection [17]. The maximum patient fluid removal rate is 1000 mL/h.

Here is the schematic for CVVH (Fig. 3.2). Notice that all pumps are accessible.

Replacement solutions in CVVH are infused into the blood circuit using replacement pump 1 through the purple line of Prismaflex set and/or the replacement pump 2 through the green line of the Prismaflex set. Replacement pump 1 infuses solution pre- or post-filter, and pump 2 infuses fluid post-filter only.

Primary therapeutic goal of CVVH is water and solute removal across a semipermeable membrane to provide fluid balance as well as control electrolyte balance. Continuous hemofiltration with the aid of a blood pump provides solute removal by convection. A replacement solution is required to drive convection [28, 93]. This type of convection utilizes no countercurrent dialysate solution (Fig. 3.2). It offers high volume ultrafiltration using replacement fluid, which can be administered pre-filter (Fig. 3.3) or post-filter (Fig. 3.4). By reducing the HCT at the blood inlet, pre-dilution is believed to reduce clotting. Post-dilution will require less replacement fluid to achieve a given clearance (dose). A combination of pre-dilution, for example, by the PBP pump, and post-dilution by the replacement pump would provide benefit in several areas and provide flexibility required to treat a given patient. Pre-dilution also means a loss between 15 and 35 % of clearance (dose), depending on the flow rates. The pump guarantees adequate blood flow to maintain required UF rates [17]. Venous blood access is usually femoral, jugular, or subclavian using a double-lumen cannula [94–96].

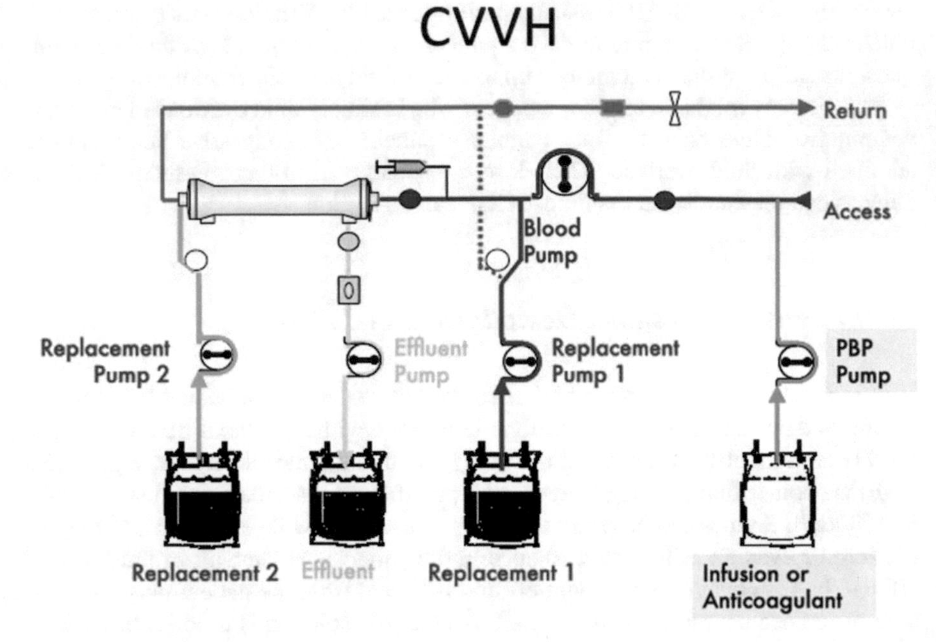

Fig. 3.2 Continuous veno-venous hemofiltration (CVVH) (Gambro Training Manual, used with permission)

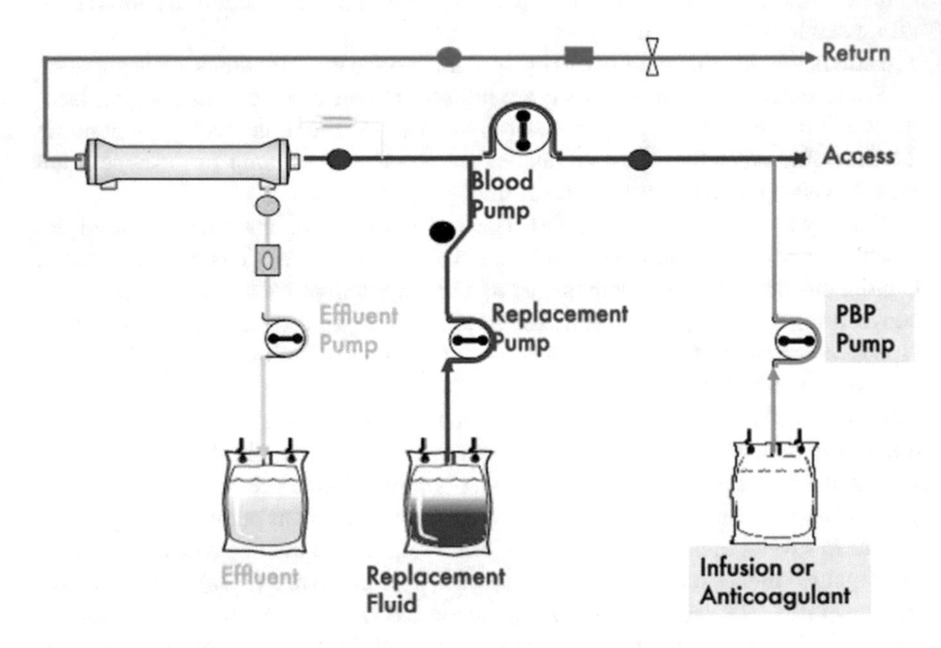

Fig. 3.3 Pre-dilution replacement solution

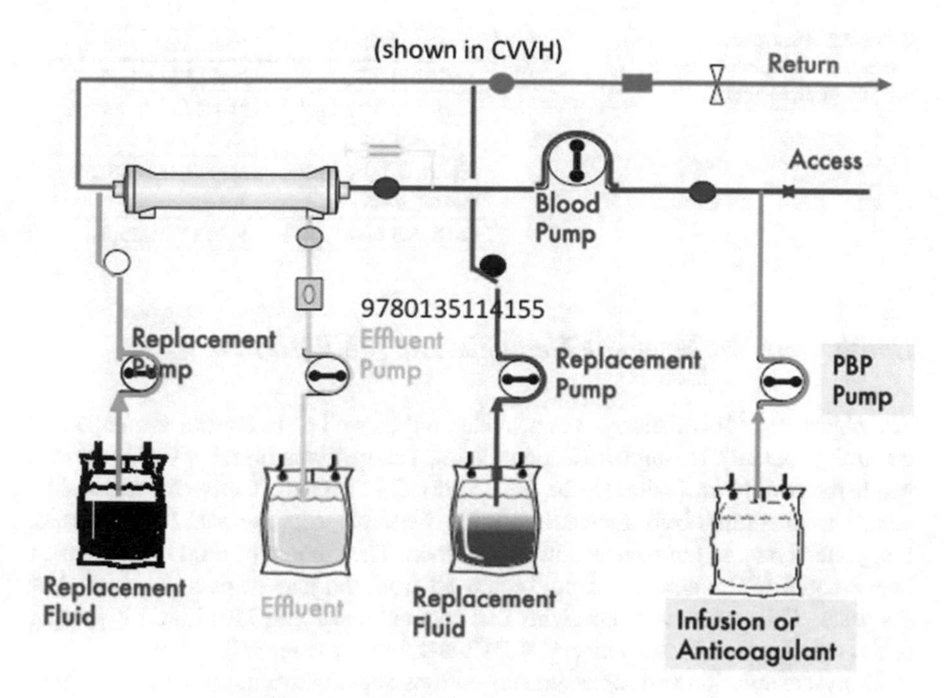

Fig. 3.4 Post-dilution replacement solution

Replacement Fluid During CVVH: Pre-filter Versus Post-filter

Replacement solutions for CVVH can be normal saline, lactated Ringer's solution, total parenteral nutrition (TPN), routine intravenous fluids, or pharmacy-made solutions (Table 3.2). Bicarbonate-buffered replacement solutions are preferred for patients with hepatic failure as patients with hepatic failure may not be able to convert lactate to bicarbonate.

Replacement fluid is given at a rate of 2000 mL/L 1.73 m^2 (35 mL/kg/h) into the circuit either before blood reaches the membrane (pre-dilution) or after passage over the filter membrane (post-dilution).

Pre-filter dilution increases the hemofilter membrane filter life. It also increases convective solute transport. Pre-filter dilution reduces solute clearance and lowers anticoagulation requirements. Some of the delivered replacement fluid will be lost by hemofiltration, thus higher ultrafiltration required given the loss of replacement fluid through filter. In post-dilution the drug clearance equals the ultrafiltration rate, while in pre-dilution the replacement fluid should be considered when calculating clearance [65, 72].

Table 3.2 Pharmacy custom-made solutions for dialysis or replacement solution

Calcium solution	Phosphorous solution
NaCl 100 mEq/L	NaCl 100 mEq/L
$NaHCO_3^-$ 35 mEq/L	$NaHCO_3^-$ 40 mEq/L
KCl 4 mEq/L	KCl 2 mEq/L
$MgSo_4$ 0.5–1.5 mEq/L	$MgSO_4$ 0.5–1.5 mEq/L
Dextrose 1.5 g/L	1.5 g/L
$CaCl_2$ 3.5 mEq/L	K_3PO_4* 2 mEq/L

Continuous Veno-venous Hemodialysis (CVVHD)

The objective of this therapy is to provide fluid as well as to control azotemia and electrolyte balance through diffusion utilizing a dialysis solution. CVVHD provides solute removal by diffusion [5, 26, 39, 74, 83]. CVVHD is effective for removal of small- to medium-sized molecules (<500 Da). No replacement fluid is used. Dialysate is pumped in counterflow to the blood. The amount of fluid in the effluent bag is equal to the amount of fluid removed from the patient plus the amount of dialysate. This schematic represents the Prismaflex set and identifies the pumps/scales that are used in the delivery of CVVHD therapy (Fig. 3.5).

Dialysate solution and replacement solutions should have the same composition to avoid staff confusion and medical errors. Many physicians are using 0.9 % saline, lactated Ringer's solution, or bicarbonate-based solutions as relatively inexpensive form of dialysate and replacement solutions that are having excessive ultrafiltration.

A dialysis solution (35–45 mL/kg/h) up to 2500 mL/m^2/h is continuously pumped through the fluid side of the filter, typically infused at 15–45 mL/min, and the concentration gradient between the filter's blood and fluid sides causes unwanted blood to diffuse into the dialysate, where they can be removed [28]. This type of dialysis utilizes diffusion solution clearance.

The total solute clearance in CRRT techniques is the sum of the convective and diffusive clearances that is the volume of effluent fluid (ultrafiltrate and dialysate). No replacement fluid is used. Convective clearance is directly proportional to the amount of filtrate produced. Small molecules are less dependent on connective clearance and are more readily removed by diffusion.

CVVHD does not use replacement fluids, but incorporates use of pumped dialysate to achieve small molecule clearance by diffusion [17, 97]. The maximum patient fluid removal rate is 1000 mL/h.

Middle- and large-size solutes such as inflammatory mediators, myoglobin, and bilirubin can be removed more efficiently by convection (CVVH) than diffusion (CVHD). The data suggest an early initiation of treatment and a minimum delivery dose of 35 mL/Kg/h improve patient survival rate [5, 8, 39, 74, 83, 87]. The minimum delivery dose of 35 mL/kg/h is the total amount of effluent, which consists of replacement solution plus patient fluid removal.

Because unwanted solutes are removed by taking off plasma water, increased clearances are achieved by using higher ultrafiltration rate to remove more plasma

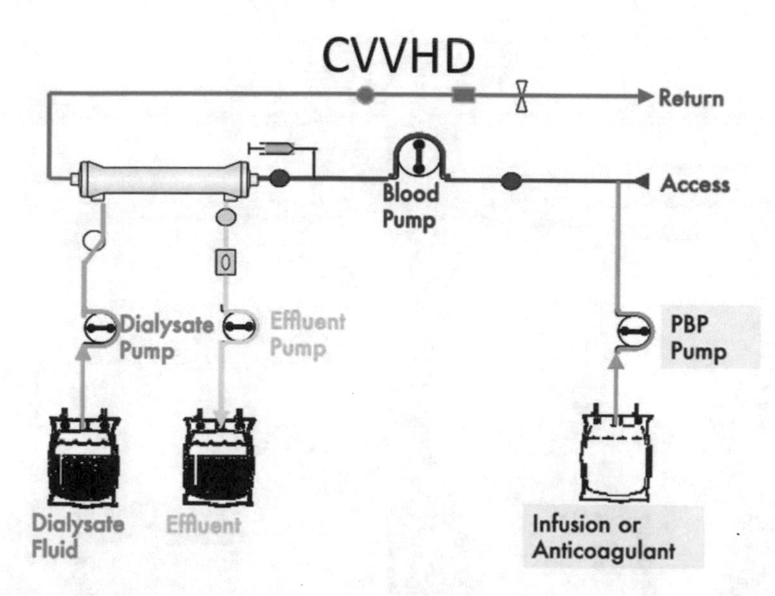

Fig. 3.5 Continuous veno-venous hemodialysis (CVVHD) (Gambro Training Manual, used with permission)

water. Compared to CVVHD therapy, CVVH provides less efficient removal of solutes of small molecular weight (<350 Da), but more efficient removal of solutes of larger molecular weight.

Continuous Veno-venous Hemodiafiltration

Continuous veno-venous hemodiafiltration (CVVHDF) combines the benefits of diffusion and convection by using both replacement fluid and dialysate.

In CVVHDF mode, all pumps can be activated. The dialysate pump functions the same as in CVVHD mode. The PBP pump functions the same as in the other modes. The replacement pump functions the same as in CVVH mode. CVVHDF mode allows the user to switch from one therapy mode to another by simply deactivating one or more solution pumps. For example, deactivating the dialysate pump would deliver CVVH; deactivating the replacement pump delivers CVVHD. The therapy delivered will be displayed on the status screen of the Prismaflex system (Fig. 3.6).

Dialysate is run on the opposite side of the filter and replacement fluid either before or after the filter. The maximum patient fluid removal rate is 1000 mL/h. CVVHD dosage is 45 mL/kg/h, ½ as dialysate and ½ as replacement fluid that can be divided into pre- and post-filter depending upon physician recommendation.

Small- and large-molecular-weight substances are both removed during CVVHDF therapy [5, 39, 74, 83]. In septic and highly catabolic patients, there is an advantage of convective over diffusive clearance [5, 39, 74].

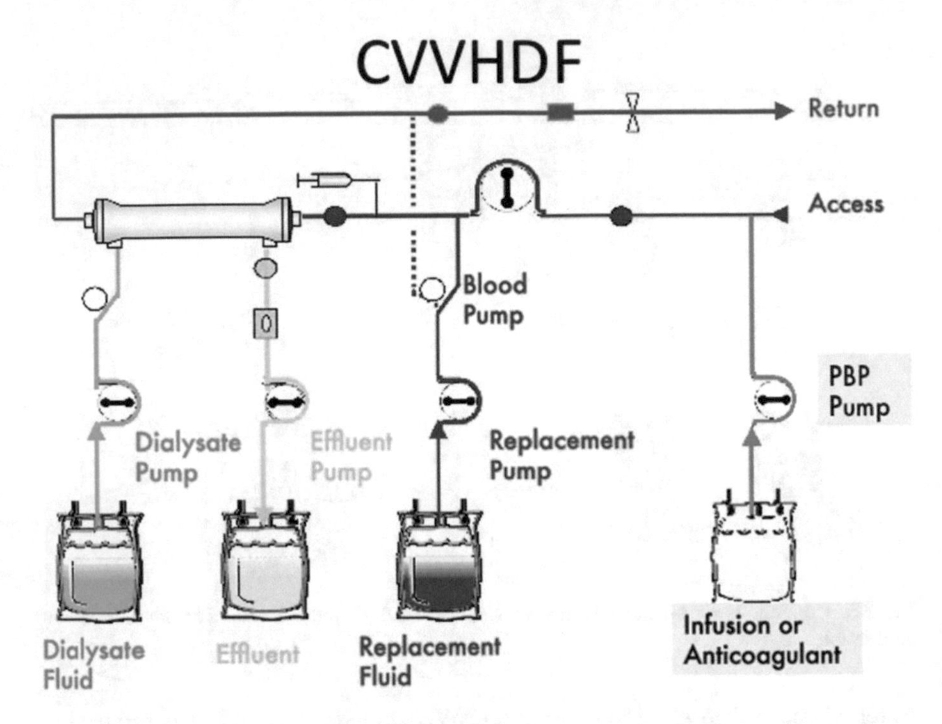

Fig. 3.6 Continuous veno-venous hemodialysis filtration (CVVHDF). It combines the benefits of CVVH and CVVHD using both convection and diffusion mechanisms (Gambro Training Manual, used with permission)

The objective of this therapy is to provide fluid and electrolyte as well as to control azotemia through both convection (replacement fluid) and diffusion (dialysate). CVVHDF combines the benefits of CVVH and CVVHD using both convective and diffusive transport mechanisms to treat any number of acute problems. It offers high volume ultrafiltration using replacement fluid, which can be administered pre-filter or post-filter. Simultaneously, dialysate is pumped in counterflow to blood. CVVHDF is a desirable therapy for patients with sepsis suffering from pro-inflammatory molecules. CVVHDF requires the use of a blood, effluent, dialysate, and replacement pumps. Both dialysate and replacement solutions are used. Plasma water and solutes are removed by diffusion, convection, and ultrafiltration. Removal of small, middle, and large molecules is achieved by diffusion and convection through the addition of dialysate solution and replacement solution, respectively. This transport mechanism is only used in CVVHDF.

Ronco's dose is 35 mL/kg/h, which is the total effluent [42, 89]. The total effluent during CVVHDF includes the spent dialysate and ultrafiltrate. Ultrafiltrate consists of replacement solution and patient fluid removal. Therefore, if you have a 35-kg patient, they require 1225 mL/h of effluent to achieve the Ronco dose. If your dialysate is set for 0.75 L/h and the patient fluid removal rate is set for 150 mL/h, then you'll have to set the replacement flow rate at 325 mL/h to achieve the Ronco dose.

Of the CRRT modalities, CVVH (connective clearance) and CVVHD (diffusion clearance) are the preferred initial therapy for children (particularly of young age and smaller size). Other factors include patients age, availability of vascular access, cardiovascular status, and nursing and technical supports.

Choosing Between the CVVH and CVVHD

Decision to use convection (hemofiltration) versus diffusion (hemodialysis) modality is based on the following factors [19]:

1. Patient's age and body weight
2. Patient's medical conditions and cardiovascular status
3. Treatment objectives with regard to fluid removal, solute removal, or both
4. Availability of vascular access
5. Supporting nursing staff and technical resources

Data has shown that CVVHD was superior to pre-dilution CVVH for clearance of urea and creatinine. Post-dilution CVVH and CVVHD gave nearly equivalent clearances [5, 26, 28, 39, 74]. In hemofiltration for sepsis, CVVH may have better cytokine clearance. Other advantages of CVVH therapy over CAVHD therapy include no minimum mean arterial pressure (MAP) required to initiate, less filter clotting due to higher blood flow, and better-controlled ultrafiltration.

CVVHD is recommended as the method of choice for the treatment of inborn errors of metabolism due to its maximal clearance of ammonium and other neurotoxicities [30, 31, 36, 37, 62, 98].

Middle- and large-size solutes such as inflammatory mediators, myoglobin, and bilirubin can be removed more efficiently by convection (CVVH) than diffusion (CVHD) [5, 39, 74]. The data suggest an early initiation of treatment and a minimum delivery dose of 35 mL/kg/h improve patient survival rate [42, 89]. The minimum delivery dose of 35 mL/kg/h is the total amount of effluent, which consists of replacement solution plus patient fluid removal.

Because unwanted solutes are removed by taking off plasma water, increased clearances are achieved by using higher ultrafiltration rate to remove more plasma water. Compared to CVVHD therapy, CVVH provides less efficient removal of solutes of small molecular weight (<350 Da), but more efficient removal of solutes of larger molecular weight.

Percent fluid overload (FO %) may be calculated as follows:

$$\text{FO}(\%) = \left[(\text{Total fluid intake}) - (\text{total fluid output}) / \text{Admission weight}\right] \times 100$$

The specific CRRT technique employed will influence the ultrafiltration rate and hence, the potential rate of drug removal. When CRRT relies solely on spontaneous blood flow without extracorporeal blood pumping, an ultrafiltration rate of 10–15 mL/min is anticipated. The addition of pumps and continuous dialysis may increase the ultrafiltration rate to 50 mL/min. Higher rates of ultrafiltration may lead to greater drug removal with a need for more frequent replacement doses. Drug removal can be determined by collection of the total volume of dialysate (ultrafiltrate) and measurement of the concentration of drug in the effluent.

Combined CRRT and Extracorporeal Membrane Oxygenation

Extracorporeal membrane oxygenation (ECMO) is a lifesaving procedure used in neonates, children, and adults with severe, reversible, cardiopulmonary failure [6, 16, 17, 48, 79]. These patients are at high risk of developing AKI and fluid overload. CRRT is commonly used to maintain fluid balance and metabolic control; however, the optimal timing, methodology, and prescriptions to support ECMO patients with renal dysfunction have not been extensively studied.

The classic CRRT indications in patients with cardiopulmonary failure on ECMO include uremia, acidosis, electrolyte abnormalities, fluid overload >10 %, and AKI (pRIFLE stage F) and the center-specific staff availability, local expertise, and experience with CRRT on ECMO currently drive decisions to initiate CRRT.

In unstable patients with multiple organ failure, ECMO can improve hemodynamic stability by increasing cardiac output and improving myocardial oxygenation. The ECMO circuit can serve as a platform for CRRT therapies. Several CRRT techniques are available to support ECMO patients with AKI and/or fluid overload. Because there are no comparison studies of these techniques, practice is based on expert opinion and local experience.

The two most common methods to provide CRRT are the use of a commercially available CRRT machine connected into the ECMO circuit or the use of an in-line hemofiltration filter into the ECMO circuit using intravenous infusion pumps to control the ultrafiltrate volume [6, 16, 17, 48, 79].

CRRT Using an In-Line Hemofilter

The introduction of a hemofiltration filter into the ECMO circuit is the most widely used method of CRRT and has the advantage of being relatively simple and inexpensive. The hemofilter is placed after the pump to provide forward blood flow and before the oxygenator to maintain the oxygenator's use as a clot and air trap in case of complications. The filter inlet is connected after the pump and the outlet is reconnected to the ECMO circuit to allow return of the blood flow to the proximal limb of the ECMO circuit. Because of the existence of a shunt, there could be a gap between the measured flow and the flow being delivered to the patient (which indicates the hemofilter blood flow rate). An ultrasonic flow probe should be placed on the arterial line of the ECMO circuit to determine the actual flow delivered to the patient.

The intravenous infusion pumps included in the circuit control the amount of replacement fluid, dialysis, and effluent fluids.

As blood comes from the patient via the venous drain cannula, it goes through the ECMO bladder to the ECMO pump, to the membrane oxygenator, and back to the patient via a return cannula. Blood is shunted from the circuit to the in-line hemofilter and returned to the ECMO pump. Fluid (ultrafiltrate) can be controlled using an intravenous pump. Replacement or dialysis fluid can be used for solute clearance and/or to achieve metabolic control.

Different combinations of the molecular clearance methods are used to achieve different CRRT modes, such as CVVH, CVVHD, CVVHDF, and SCUF. There are several methods to determine the amount of fluid being removed. One possible method is to assume that the fluid delivered/removed is equal to the rate of the infusion pumps. This assumption may be inaccurate as the infusion pumps are actually flow restrictors.

Measuring the actual volume of the ultrafiltrate removed by weight or using a volumetric measuring device could be the most precise method. However, this requires strict control by the nursing staff and an inevitable increase in the nursing workload. Another defect is the absence of pressure monitoring in the hemofiltration circuit, which may lead to delayed detection of clotting or rupture of the filter. No additional regional anticoagulation is needed since the patient and the entire circuit is already heparinized for ECMO. Circuit for the CRRT can usually be saline due to the relative small size of CRRT circuit in ratio to the larger ECMO circuit.

CRRT Using a CRRT Machine

In this method, the CRRT machine is typically connected to the venous limb of the roller-head ECMO circuit before the pump. The blood is then returned from the CRRT machine to the ECMO circuit near the venous CRRT connection and before the ECMO pump.

If a centrifugal ECMO pump is used, the CRRT machine should not be placed before the ECMO pump because there is a very risk of air entrainment. Instead, the CRRT machine should be placed after the ECMO bladder to prevent air entrapment. Dialysis or replacement fluid (pre-filter or post-filter) is used to efficiently clear solutes, and ultrafiltrate can be generated to remove the desired fluid.

If the ECMO circuit uses a roller pump, a proportion of the circuit blood comes from the patient via the venous drain cannula and enters the RRT machine where replacement, dialysis, and ultrafiltration occur. Blood from the RRT machine then goes back to the ECMO bladder to the ECMO pump, the membrane oxygenator, and back to the patient via a return cannula.

CRRT Solutions

Replacement Solutions

Replacement solutions are used to increase the amount of convective solute removal in CVVH and CVVHDF [20, 35, 53]. Typical replacement fluid rates are 1000–2000 mL/h. Physicians prescribe replacement solution up to 4500 mL/h. Fluid composition is dependent on patient status and adjusted accordingly. Route of administration, either pre- or post-filter, is also prescribed (Fig. 2.2).

Pre-filter replacement increases filter life, reduces solute clearance, and lowers anticoagulation requirements.

Replacement solutions for CVVH often contain electrolytes and buffer. The amount of electrolytes approximates to physiologic levels, unless trying to adjust the patient's serum level. The following electrolyte ranges are used during CRRT (mEq/L): Na 117–132, K 0–4, Cl 95–110, calcium 0–3.5, and Mg 0.75–1.5. Bicarbonate is the preferred buffer to normalize serum pH during CRRT since it is physiologic [89, 91, 98–100]. Bicarbonate levels may approximate to physiologic levels or not, depending on the patient's needs, with range being 22–35 mEq/L. Lactate is not desirable as a buffer during CVVH because it results in elevated serum lactate levels; however, some physicians still prescribe it [91, 93, 99, 101, 102].

Replacement fluids may be administered pre- or post-filter. Replacement solution is removed at the same rate it was infused, which can cause hemoconcentration and filter clotting. Pre-filter replacement fluids are often referred to as "pre-dilution" fluids. The effluent fluid removal rate (35 mL/kg/h) = ultrafiltration + replacement fluid.

Both lactate- and the bicarbonate-based solutions result in the same degree of effective clearance, but plasma lactate levels are higher in patients on lactate-based solutions [91, 93, 99, 101, 102]. Elevated lactate levels may offer serious adverse effects in the setting of sepsis and/or organ under-perfusion.

Furthermore, patients with hepatic failure may not be able to convert lactate to bicarbonate, and the use of lactate-based dialysis solution may produce or exacerbate lactic acidosis. Bicarbonate-buffered dialysis solutions are therefore preferred for patients with hepatic failure. Essentially with the use of these products, the use of lactate- based solutions should be considered historical and potentially detrimental to the child needing CRRT.

Solutions for CVVH can be as uncomplicated as normal saline, lactated Ringer's solution, total parenteral nutrition (TPN), routine intravenous fluids, or pharmacy-made solutions (Table 3.2) or compounded solutions (Normocarb®) [91, 93, 101]. Many programs will use saline or lactated Ringer's solution as a relatively inexpensive form of replacement fluid in those patients who are having excessive ultrafiltration.

The decision to use replacement fluid is often based on the overall solute and ultrafiltration clearance requirements of the patient as well as the local standard of care.

Dialysis solutions are also available both in lactate and bicarbonate forms.

Additionally, pharmacy-made or pharmacy-customized solutions (usually bicarbonate based) are also available. Further Normocarb® and PrismaSATE BGK 2/0 are calcium-free dialysate solutions, providing a venue for the provision of either citrate or alternate anticoagulation.

Replacement solution infused into the blood prior to the blood entering the filter will dilute the blood and reduce hemoconcentration inside the filter. This could increase your filter life, but provide less efficient solute removal than if you infuse replacement solution post-filter.

Dialysate Solutions

Ronco treated an infant for the first time in 1980 with continuous arteriovenous hemofiltration (CAVH) [7]. The standard dialysate composition (PrismaSATE) is as follows: (mEq/L) Na 140, K 0 mEq, Cl 109.5, Ca 3.5, Mg 1.0, lactate 3 mEq (if using lactate-buffered solution) and bicarbonate 32 mEq (if using bicarbonate solution), and glucose 0 mg (Table 3.2).

Electrolyte concentrations may be adjusted per individual need. Lactate buffer may be problematic especially in patients with liver involvement. Peritoneal dialysis solutions are very high in glucose, increasing insulin requirement, and should not be used (Table 3.2).

Through diffusion, dialysate corrects underlying metabolic problems. Dialysate effectiveness is dependent on its buffering agent, electrolytes, and glucose contents. Dialysate formulas should reflect normal plasma values to achieve homeostasis. Bicarbonate-based solutions are physiologic and replace lost bicarbonate immediately without the risk of alkalosis and improve hemodynamic stability with fewer cardiovascular events. Bicarbonate-based solutions are the preferred buffer for patients with compromised liver function [91, 93, 101].

Lactate, in the lactic-based solution, is converted in the liver, under normal conditions, on a 1:1 basis to bicarbonate and can sufficiently correct acidosis. Lactate-based solutions, however, have an acid pH value of 5.4, are a powerful peripheral vasodilator, and may cause further acidosis for patients with hypoxia, liver failure, and those with preexisting lactic acidosis.

Vascular Access and Catheter Size

Access to blood supply for the extra corporeal circuit varies with CRRT techniques. Arteriovenous techniques, which have largely fallen out of favor, generally require cannulation of the femoral artery and the femoral vein.

A properly functioning vascular access is needed to provide adequate blood flow for patients receiving CRRT. Vascular access for CRRT most often is accomplished by placement of a dialysis catheter in the right internal jugular or femoral vein [94–96, 103]. This is due to the fact that as the child "wiggles," there will be less effect of blood flow rate with a "high" line as opposed to a "low" line. All access is preferred to be placed in the right internal jugular vein if possible due to the effect on patient care, turning in bed, and flexing the legs, all of which affect blood flow rate [94–96, 103]. Further, the size of the blood vessel in the cardiac region is larger, allowing for larger access. The final reason why an internal jugular is preferred is that as the child recovers, the child can ambulate without risk of bending a femoral placed catheter. The subclavian vein catheter should be avoided because of its potential for kinking and the high risk of venous stenosis [94–96, 103]. The variable blood flow rates lead to a higher risk of thrombosis. In general, large bore, small length catheters are preferable for CRRT procedures to permit a high blood flow rate. In pumped (veno-venous) systems, double-lumen venous catheters are commonly used; the size should be selected based on the site of insertion to optimize flow.

Blood recirculation from the venous to the arterial port can reduce the effectiveness of dialytic therapies, particularly during intermittent hemodialysis.

Ideal catheter characteristics are the catheters with large internal diameter and short length to minimize resistance and to allow adequate blood flow without vessel damage (Table 3.3). Match catheter size to patient size and anatomical site. Minimum blood flow rate of 30–50 mL/min is required to minimize access and filter clotting (neonates and infants 10–12 mL/kg/min; 4–6 mL/kg/min in children; 2–5 mL/kg/min in adolescents). Use of a short catheter in the femoral vein with high efficiency dialysis may result in up to 23 % blood flow recirculation and can be avoided by using longer catheters when using the femoral vein for vascular access [96].

Uncuffed double-lumen dialysis catheters can be used at the bedside. The catheter size for acute dialysis is shown in Table 3.2 [96]. To avoid the chances of clotting, it is recommended to maintain optimal blood flow rate in the extracorporeal circuit and install heparin lock (1000–5000 U/mL) into the catheter.

Monitoring

Patient must be continuously monitored during CRR for circuit patency, blood pressure, hemodynamic stability, level of consciousness, acid–base and electrolytes balance, hematological status, infection, nutritional status, air embolus, blood flow rate, ultrafiltration flow rate, dialysate/replacement flow rate, and ultrafiltrate/filter leak.

Table 3.3 Suggested size and location of vascular access based upon size of the child[a]

Patient size	Catheter size and source	Site of insertion
NEONATE	Dual-lumen 5.0–7.0 French (COOK/MEDCOMP)	Umbilical, internal/external-jugular, or femoral vein subclavian or femoral vein
3–6 kg	Dual-lumen 7.0 French (COOK/MEDCOMP)	Internal/external-jugular, subclavian or femoral vein
6–15 kg	Dual-lumen 8.0 French (KENDALL, ARROW)	Internal/external-jugular, subclavian or femoral vein
15–30 kg	Dual-lumen 9.0 French (MEDCOMP)	Internal/external-jugular, subclavian or femoral vein
>30 kg	Dual-lumen 10.0–12.5 French (ARROW, KENDALL)	Internal/external-jugular, subclavian or femoral vein

[a]References [94–96, 103]

CRRT can be performed for several days to few weeks. Careful monitoring of blood chemistries is required every 12–24 h. An hourly net UF rate must be recorded and kept at the bedside. Clotting of the filter and bleeding particularly in the postoperative patient infection are the major complications of CRRT.

CRRT Machinery

All newer commercially available CRRT machines have a variety of blood flow rate (BFR), a blood pump segment with air leak detector, a heater, warming systems, accurate ultrafiltration controllers, venous and arterial pressure monitors, and blood leak detectors. When blood is outside of the body, a tremendous heat loss occurs. Additional overhead warmer or external warmer may be needed. Remember it is rare to "spike a temp" on hemofiltration; therefore, attention to signs of sepsis is needed, for temperature spikes will not occur.

The Baxter, Gambro, Braun, and Fresenius machines allow for individual choice of hemofilter membrane, while the PRISMA (Gambro) uses a prefixed membrane (AN-69) with two surface areas (M60 0.6 m^2 and M60 0.9 m^2) [67]. In addition to rigidity of prescription and performance, PRISMA machine comes with a predesigned circuit with either pre- or post-dilution or no interchange of therapy possible. The blood flow is also limited to 180 mL/min. The choice of CRRT machine is based on the local standard of care as opposed to clinical outcome.

A dedicated neonatal CRRT machine, the Cardio–Renal Pediatric Dialysis Emergency Machine (CARPEDIEM), comes with polysulfone membranes; surface areas of 0.07, 0.147, and 0.245 m^2 with small circuit volume of 27.2, 33.5; and 41.5 mL and blood pump flow rate of 5–50 mL/min (Fig. 3.7) [75]. It provides maximum total ultrafiltration/dialysis/hemofiltration of as little as 5 mL/min.

Extracorporeal Blood Volume

Low extracorporeal blood volume is essential. The extracorporeal blood volume should be maintained at 8–10 % of the patient's blood volume with the use of appropriate size of catheters, small hemofilters, and small tubing set volume. Blood tubing priming volumes in children vary from 25 mL for neonatal catheter to 75 mL for pediatric size catheter. Priming of the circuit should be with normal saline. If the extracorporeal volume is greater than 10 % of the patient's total blood volume, blood or 5 % albumin should be used to priming the circuit. In the anemic and hypotensive child, the circuit may require priming with packed red cells before starting CRRT. The total body volume is about 100 mL/kg of body weight in neonates and 80 mL/kg of body weight in infants and children.

Small tubing set and filter should be also used to minimize clotting. A M60 set is 93 mL extracorporeal volume including filter and bloodlines (SA $\geq$0.6 m^2) and is considered as a good hemofilter for diffuse mode use for patients $\leq$50 kg weight.

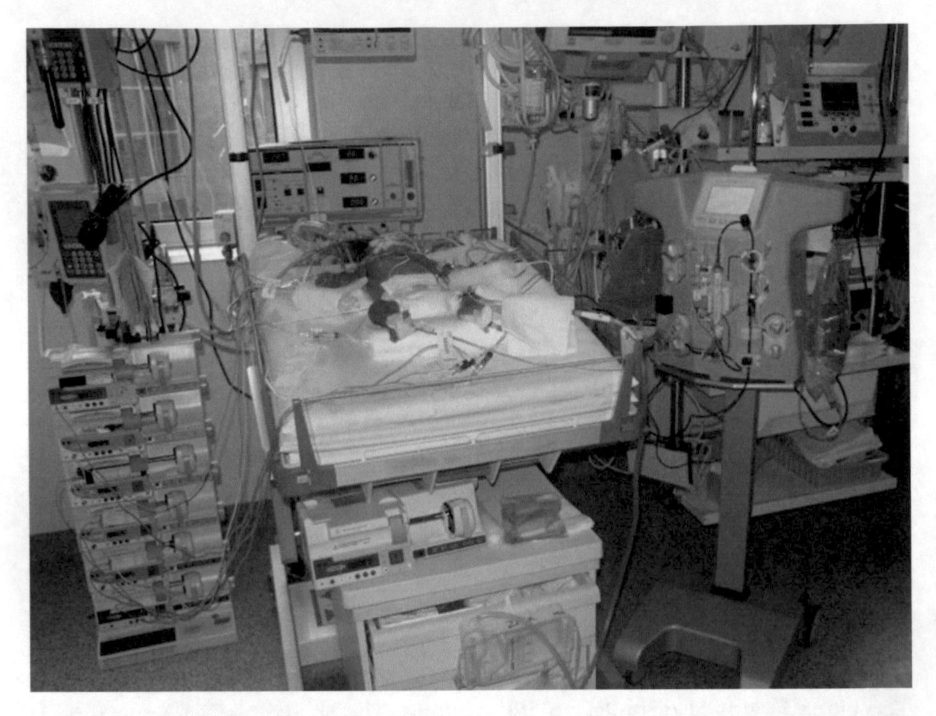

Fig. 3.7 Cardio-Renal Pediatric Dialysis Emergency Machine (CARPEDIEM)

The use of AN69 polyacrylonitrile membrane in children may cause bradykinin release syndrome when a blood prime has been used. The bradykinin release syndrome is a steep decline in blood pressure after the initiation of CRRT when the blood is exposed to the highly negatively charged AN69. Buffering the blood to physiologic pH before priming the circuit or infusing the blood post-filter at the same rate as a saline prime can prevent this problem with the use of a priming mixture of 50 mL PRBC, 50 mL sodium bicarbonate, and 45 mg calcium chloride.

Intravascular Blood Volume Determination

Weight	cc/kg
Neonates	100
≤10 kg	80
>10 kg	70

Therefore, a 20 kg child has 1.4 L intravascular blood volume.

Hemofilter Membrane

Hemofilter membranes (polysulfone, AN-69, AN-69 ST) are composed of high-flux synthetic/biocompatible material. Structural design is characterized by high fluid removal and molecular cutoff weight of 30,000–50,000 Da. The semipermeable membranes provide an interface between the blood and dialysate compartment. Biocompatibility minimizes severe patient reactions and decreases the complement activation [67].

The use of more biocompatible membranes (AN-69 polyacrylonitrile) results in less complement activation. Hemodialysis data has shown that biocompatible membranes improve survival in AKI, have a shorter time to recovery of renal function, and are less associated with oliguria. However, AN-69 membranes have been associated with "bradykinin release syndrome" in patients on ACE inhibitors. This "bradykinin release syndrome" is pH dependent. Buffering the blood with THAM, calcium chloride, or sodium bicarbonate and bypassing the membrane (priming circuit with saline and run packed red blood cell into patient on venous return line have been shown to be effective in minimizing membrane reaction). Alternative to the AN-69 membrane, AN-69 ST (surface treated) membrane can be used in acidotic membrane situations in retarding or minimizing membrane reaction.

Generally speaking, the efficiency of small solute clearance in CRRT is largely determined by dialysate/ultrafiltration flow rate; therefore, solute removal characteristics are not an important factor in choosing a dialysis membrane.

High-flux membranes, which are designed to provide high water permeability, are generally recommended for hemofiltration procedures. Finally, although there is no conclusive evidence that membrane biocompatibility affects patient outcome, there is general consensus that the use of synthetic membranes is preferable over cellulose-based membranes for the treatment of patients with AKI. The choice of membrane is usually linked to the choice of CRRT machine. AN-69 may be superior in sepsis.

References

1. Brophy PD, Maxvold NJ, Bunchman TE. CAVH/CVVH in pediatric patients. In: Nissenson AR, Fine RN, editors. Dialysis. 3rd ed. Philadelphia: Hanley & Belfus; 2002.
2. Goldstein SL, Somers MJ, Brophy PD, et al. The prospective pediatric continuous renal replacement therapy (ppCRRT) registry: design, development and data assessed. Int J Artif Organs. 2004;27(1):9–14.
3. Gottlieb R, Assadi F. Continuous renal replacement therapy in newborn infants. In: Spitzer AR, editor. Intensive care of the fetus and neonate. Philadelphia: Mosby-Year Book; 1995. p. 1187–91.
4. Paganini E, O'Hara P, Nakamoto S. Slow continuous ultrafiltration in hemodialysis resistant oliguric renal failure. Trans Am Soc Artif Intern Organs. 1984;30:173–8.
5. Parakininkas D, Greenbaum LA. Comparison of solute clearance in three modes of continuous renal replacement therapy. Pediatr Crit Care Med. 2004;5(3):269–74.

6. Ricci Z, Ronco C, Picardo S. CRRT in series with extracorporeal membrane oxygenation in pediatric patients. Kidney Int. 2010;77(5):469–70.
7. Ronco C, Lauer A, Saccaggi A, Belledonne M, Glabman S, Bosch JP. Continuous arteriovenous hemofiltration in the critically ill patient. Clinical use and operational characteristics. Ann Intern Med. 1983;99(4):445–60.
8. Roy D, Hogg RJ, Wilby PA, et al. Continuous veno-venous hemodiafiltration using bicarbonate dialysate. Pediatr Nephrol. 1997;11(6):680–3.
9. Sutherland SM, Alexander SR. Continuous renal replacement therapy in children. Pediatr Nephrol. 2012;27:2007–16.
10. Van de Kerkhove MP, Poyck PP, Deurholt T, et al. Liver support therapy: an overview of the AMC-bioartificial liver research. Dig Surg. 2005;22(4):254–64.
11. Wigg AJ, Padbury RT. Liver support systems: promise and reality. Gastroenterol Hepatol. 2005;20(12):1807–16.
12. Zhang YL, Hu WP, Zhou LH, Wang Y, Cheng A, Shao SN, Hon LL, Chen QY. Continuous renal replacement therapy in children with multiple organ dysfunction syndrome: a case series. Int Braz J Urol. 2014;40(6):846–52.
13. Ronco C, Pohlmeier R, Tetta C. Intermittent or continuous treatment of acute renal failure? Crit Care Med. 2003;31(9):2417.
14. Auron A, Brophy PD. Pediatric renal supportive therapies: the changing face of pediatric renal replacement approaches. Curr Opin Pediatr. 2010;22:183–8.
15. Bunchman TE. Treatment of acute kidney injury in children: from conservative management to renal replacement therapy. Nat Clin Pract Nephrol. 2008;4:510–4.
16. Chen H, Yu RG, Yin NN, Zhou JA. Combination of extracorporeal membrane oxygenation and continuous renal replacement therapy in critically ill patients: a systemic review. Crit Care. 2014;18(6):675.
17. Clark WR, Mueller B, Kraus A, et al. Extracorporeal therapy requirements for patients with acute renal failure. J Am Soc Nephrol. 1997;8:804–12.
18. Dialysis Working Group. Renal replacement therapy for acute renal failure in children: European guidelines. Pediatr Nephrol. 2004;19(2):199–207.
19. Flynn JT. Choice of dialysis modality for management of pediatric acute renal failure. Pediatr Nephrol. 2002;17:61–9.
20. Goldstein SL. Overview of pediatric renal replacement therapy in acute kidney injury. Semin Dial. 2009;22:180–4.
21. Hsu RK, McCulloch CE, Dudley RA, et al. Temporal changes in incidence of dialysis-requiring AKI. J Am Soc Nephrol. 2012;24:37–42.
22. Joy MS, Matzke GR, Armstrong DK, Marx MA, Zarowitz BJ. A primer on continuous renal replacement therapy for critically ill patients. Ann Pharmacother. 1998;32:362–75.
23. Kellum JA, Angus DC, Johnson JP, et al. Continuous versus intermittent renal replacement therapy: a meta-analysis. Intensive Care Med. 2002;28:29–37.
24. Maxvold NJ, Smoyer WE, Custer JR, Bunchman TE. Amino acid loss and nitrogen balance in critically ill children with acute renal failure: a comparison between CVVH and CVVHD therapies. Crit Care Med. 2000;28:1161–5.
25. Mehta RL, Letteri JM. Current status of renal replacement therapy for acute renal failure. A survey of US nephrologists. Am J Nephrol. 1999;19:377–82.
26. Bellomo R. Choosing a therapeutic modality: hemofiltration vs. hemodialysis vs. hemodiafiltration. Semin Dial. 1996;9:88–92.
27. Boschee ED, Cave DA, Garros D, Lequier L, Granoski DA, Guerra GG, et al. Indications and outcomes in children receiving renal replacement therapy in pediatric intensive care. J Crit Care. 2014;29:37–42.
28. Brunet S, Leblanc M, Geadah D, et al. Diffusive and convective solute clearances during continuous renal replacement therapy at various dialysate and ultrafiltration flow rates. Am J Kidney Dis. 1999;34:486–92.

29. Bunchman TE, Brophy PD, Goldstein SL. Technical considerations for renal replacement therapy in children. Semin Nephrol. 2008;28:488–92.
30. Bunchman TE, Ferris ME. Management of toxic ingestions with the use of renal replacement therapy. Pediatr Nephrol. 2011;26:535–41.
31. Deodato F, Boenzi S, Rizzo C, et al. Inborn errors of metabolism: an update on epidemiology and on neonatal-onset hyperammonemia. Acta Paediatr Suppl. 2004;93(445):18–21.
32. Fleming GM, Walters S, Goldstein SL, Alexander SR, Baum MA, Blowey DL, et al. Nonrenal indications for continuous renal replacement therapy: a report from the prospective pediatric continuous renal replacement therapy registry group. Pediatr Crit Care. 2012;13:e299–304.
33. Foland JA, Fortenberry JD, Warshaw BL, et al. Fluid over load before continuous hemofiltration and survival in critically ill children: a retrospective analysis. Crit Care Med. 2004;32(8):1771–6.
34. Gillespie RS, Seidel K, Symons JM. Effect of fluid overload and dose of replacement fluid on survival in hemofiltration. Pediatr Nephrol. 2004;19(12):1394–9.
35. Goldstein SL. Continuous renal replacement therapy: mechanism of clearance, fluid removal, indications and outcomes. Curr Opin Pediatr. 2011;23:181–5.
36. Kim HJ, Park SL, Park KI, Lee JS, Eun HS, Kim JH, et al. Acute treatment of hyperammonemia by continuous renal replacement therapy in a newborn patient with ornithine transcarbamylase deficiency. Korean J Pediatr. 2011;54(10):425–8.
37. McBryde KD, Kershaw DB, Bunchman TE, et al. Renal replacement therapy in the treatment of confirmed or suspected inborn errors of metabolism. J Pediatr. 2006;148(6):770–8.
38. Schetz M. Non-renal indications for continuous renal replacement therapy. Kidney Int Suppl. 1999;72:S88–94.
39. Siegler MH, Teehan BP. Solute transport in continuous hemodialysis: a new treatment for acute renal failure. Kidney Int. 1987;32:562–71.
40. Silvester W. Mediator removal with CRRT: complement and cytokines. Am J Kidney Dis. 1997;30(5 Suppl 4):S38–43.
41. Sutherland SM, Zappitelli M, Alexander SR, Chua AN, Brophy PD, Bunchman TE, et al. Fluid overload and mortality in children receiving continuous renal replacement therapy: the prospective pediatric continuous renal replacement therapy registry. Am J Kidney Dis. 2010;55(2):316–25.
42. Ronco C, Ricci Z. Pediatric continuous renal replacement: 20 years later. Intensive Care Med. 2015;41(6):985–93.
43. Ronco C, Ricci Z, Goldstein SL. Revolution in the management of acute kidney injury in newborns. Am J Kidney Dis. 2015; May 7. Pil:S0272(15)00620-4. doi:10.1053/J.ajkd.2015.03.029 [Epub ahead of print].
44. Santiago MJ, Lopez-Herce J, Urbano J, del Castillo J, Sanchez A, Bellon JM, et al. Continuous renal replacement therapy in children after cardiac surgery. J Thorac Cardiovasc Surg. 2013;146(2):448–54.
45. Kellum JA, Mehta RL, Angus DC, et al. The first international consensus conference on continuous renal replacement therapy. Kidney Int. 2002;62:1855–63.
46. Korneckki A, Tauman R, Lubetzky R, Sivan Y. Continuous renal replacement therapy for non-renal indications: experience in children. Isr Med Assoc J. 2002;4(5):345–8.
47. Meyer TW, Walther JL, Pagtalunan ME, et al. The clearance of protein bound solutes by hemofiltration and hemodiafiltration. Kidney Int. 2005;68(2):867–77.
48. Askenazi DJ, Selewski DT, Paden ML, Cooper DS, Bridges BC, Zappitelli M, et al. Renal replacement therapy in critically ill patients receiving extracorporeal membrane oxygenation. Clin J Am Soc Nephrol. 2012;7(8):1328–36.
49. Bunchman TE. Fluid overload in multiple organ dysfunction syndrome: a prediction of survival. Crit Care Med. 2004;32(8):1805–6.
50. Cole L, Bellomo R, Hart G, et al. A phase II randomized, controlled trial of continuous hemofiltration in sepsis. Crit Care Med. 2002;30:100–6.

51. Davenport A, Will E, Davidson A. Improved cardiovascular stability during continuous modes of renal replacement therapy in critically ill patients with acute hepatic and renal failure. Crit Care Med. 1993;21:328–38.
52. Elahi MM, Lim MY, Joseph RN, et al. Early hemofiltration improves survival in post-cardiotomy patients with acute renal failure. Eur J Cardiothorac Surg. 2004;26(5):1027–31.
53. Goldstein SL. Advances in pediatric renal replacement therapy for acute kidney injury. Semin Dial. 2011;24(2):187–91.
54. Goldstein SL, Somers MJ, Baum M, et al. Pediatric patients with multi-organ system failure receiving continuous renal replacement therapy. Kidney Int. 2005;67(2):653–8.
55. Golper TA. Continuous arteriovenous hemofiltration in acute renal failure. Am J Kidney Dis. 1985;6(6):373–86.
56. Bouman CS, Oudemans-Van Straaten HM, Tissen JG, Zandstra DF, Kesecioglu J. Effect of early high-volume continuous venovenous hemofiltration on survival and recovery of renal function in intensive care patients with acute renal failure: a prospective, randomized trial. Crit Care Med. 2002;30(10):2205–11.
57. DiCarlo JV, Alexander SR, Agarwal R, Schiffman JD. Continuous veno-venous hemofiltration may improve survival from acute respiratory distress syndrome after bone marrow transplantation or chemotherapy. J Pediatr Hematol Oncol. 2003;25(10):801–5.
58. Flores FX, Brophy PD, Symons JM, Fortenberry JD, Chua AN, Alexander S, et al. Continuous renal replacement therapy after stem cell transplantation. A report from the prospective pediatric CRRT registry group. Pediatr Nephrol. 2008;23(4):625–30.
59. Maxvold NJ, Bunchman TE. Renal failure and renal replacement therapy. Crit Care Clin. 2003;19(3):563–75.
60. McDonald BR, Mehta RL. Transmembrane flux of IL-1B and TNF-alpha in patients undergoing continuous arteriovenous hemodialysis (CAVHD). J Am Soc Nephrol. 1990;1:3.68–71.
61. Meyer RJ, Brophy PD, Bunchman TE, et al. Survival and renal function in pediatric patients following extracorporeal life support with hemofiltration. Pediatr Crit Care Med. 2001;2:238–42.
62. Naruse K. Artificial liver support: future aspects. J Artif Organs. 2005;8(2):71–6.
63. Symons JM, Brophy PD, Gregory MJ, et al. Continuous renal replacement therapy in children up to 10 kg. Am J Kidney Dis. 2003;41(5):984–9.
64. Zobel G, Kuttnig M, Ring E, Grubbauer HM. Clinical scoring systems in children with continuous extracorporeal renal support. Child Nephrol Urol. 1990;10:14–7.
65. Grootendorst AF, Van Bommel EFH, Van Der Hoven B, et al. High-volume hemofiltration improves hemodynamics of endotoxin-induced shock in the pig. J Crit Care. 1992;7:67–75.
66. Hackbarth RM, Eding D, Gianoli-Smith C, et al. Zero balance ultrafiltration (Z-BUF) in blood-primed CRRT circuits achieves electrolyte and acid-base homeostasis prior to patient connection. Pediatr Nephrol. 2005;20(9):1328–33.
67. Lacour F, Maheut H. AN-69 membrane and conversion enzyme inhibitors: prevention of anaphylactic shock by alkaline rinsing? Nephrologie. 1992;13(3):135–6.
68. Macias WA, Clark WR. Acid base balance in continuous renal replacement therapy. Semin Dial. 1996;9:145–51.
69. Bunchman TE, Maxvold NJ, Kershaw DB, et al. Continuous veno-venous hemodiafiltration in infants and children. Pediatr Nephrol. 1994;8:96–9.
70. Burchardi H. Renal replacement therapy (RRT) in the ICU: criteria for initiating RRT. In: Ronco C, Bellomo R, La Greca G, editors. Blood purification in intensive care (Contributions to Nephrology V 132- Berlyne GM and Ronco C). New York: Karger; 2001. p. 171–80.
71. Garzotto F, Zanella M, Ronco C. The evolution of pediatric continuous renal replacement therapy. Nephron Clin Pract. 2014;127(1–4):172–5.
72. Jiang HL, Xue WJ, Li DQ, et al. Pre- vs. post-dilution CVVH. Blood Purif. 2005;23(4):338.
73. Kara OD, Dincel N, Kaplan Bulut I, Yilmaz E, Ozdemir K, Gozuoglu G, et al. Success of continuous veno-venous hemofiltration in children monitored in the intensive care units. Ren Fail. 2014;36(9):1411–5.
74. Ronco C, Tetta C, Mariano F, et al. Interpreting the mechanisms of continuous renal replacement therapy in sepsis: the peak concentration hypothesis. Artif Organs. 2003;27(9):792–801.

75. Ronco C, Garzotto F, Brendolan A, Zanella M, Bellettato M, Vedovato S, et al. Continuous renal replacement therapy in neonates and small infants: development and use of a miniaturised machine (CARPEDIEM). Lancet. 2014;383(9931):1807–13.
76. Tonelli M, Manns B, Feller-Kopman D. Acute renal failure in the intensive care unit: a systematic review of the impact of dialytic modality or mortality and renal recovery. Am J Kidney Dis. 2002;40:875–85.
77. Pannu N, Gibney RN. Renal replacement therapy in the intensive care unit. Ther Clin Risk Manag. 2005;1:141–50.
78. Parekh RS, Bunchman TE. Dialysis support in the pediatric intensive care unit. Adv Ren Replace Ther. 1996;3:326–36.
79. Picca S, Dionisi-Vici C, Abeni D, et al. Extracorporeal dialysis in neonatal hyperammonemia: modalities and prognostic indicators. Pediatr Nephrol. 2001;16(11):862–7.
80. Piccinni P, Dan M, Barbacini S, et al. Early isovolaemic haemofiltration in oliguric patients with septic shock. Intensive Care Med. 2006;32(1):80–6.
81. Assadi F. Treatment of acute renal failure in an infant by continuous arteriovenous hemodialysis. Pediatr Nephrol. 1988;2:230–2.
82. Baird JS, Wald EL. Long-term (>4 weeks) continuous renal replacement therapy in critical illness. Int J Artif Organs. 2010;33(10):716–20.
83. Lee CY, Yeh HC, Lin CY. Treatment of critically ill children with kidney injury by sustained low-efficiency daily diafiltration. Pediatr Nephrol. 2012;27:2301–9.
84. Mehta RL, McDonald B, Gabbai FB, et al. A randomized clinical trial of continuous versus intermittent dialysis for acute renal failure. Kidney Int. 2001;60(3):1154–63.
85. Ponikvar R, Kandus A, Urbancic A, Kornhauser AG, Primozic J, Ponikvar JB. Continuous renal replacement therapy and plasma exchange in newborns and infants. Artif Organs. 2002;26:163–8.
86. Ronco C, Parenzan L. Acute renal failure in infancy: treatment by continuous renal replacement therapy. Intensive Care Med. 1995;21:490–9.
87. Warady B, Bunchman T. Dialysis therapy for children with acute renal failure: survey results. Pediatr Nephrol. 2000;15:11–3.
88. Gibney N, Hoste E, Burdmann EA, Bunchman T, Kher V, Viswanathan R, et al. Timing of initiation and discontinuation of renal replacement therapy in AKI: unanswered key questions. Clin J Am Soc Nephrol. 2008;3:876–80.
89. Ronco C, Belomo R, Homel P, et al. Effects of different doses in continuous venovenous hemofiltration on outcomes of acute renal failure: a prospective randomized trial. Lancet. 2000;356:26–30.
90. Askenazi DJ, Goldstein MD, Koralkar R, Fortenberry MD, Baum M, et al. Continuous renal replacement therapy for children ≤10 kg: a report from the prospective pediatric continuous renal replacement therapy registry. J Pediatr. 2013;162:587–92.
91. Zimmerman D, Cotman P, Ting R, et al. Continuous veno-venous haemodialysis with a novel bicarbonate dialysis solution: prospective cross-over comparison with a lactate buggered solution. Nephrol Dial Transplant. 1999;14:2387–91.
92. McBryde KD, Kudelka TL, Kershaw DB, et al. Clearance of amino acids by hemodialysis in argininosuccinate synthetase deficiency. J Pediatr. 2004;144(4):536–40.
93. Bunchman TE, Maxvold NJ, Brophy PD. Pediatric convective hemofiltration: Normocarb® replacement fluid and citrate anticoagulation. Am J Kidney Dis. 2003;42(6):1248–52.
94. Bunchman TE. Wilson SE (ed): Vascular access: principles and practice, 4th ed Mosby, St. Louis, 2002. Pediatr Nephrol. 2003;18(9):968.
95. Hackbarth R, Bunchman TE, Chue AN, et al. The effect of vascular access location and size on circuit survival in pediatric continuous renal support therapy: a report from the PCRRT registry. Int J Artif Organs. 2007;30:1116–21.
96. Jenkins RD, Kuhn RJ, Funk JE. Clinical implications of catheter variability on neonatal continuous hemofiltration. Trans Am Soc Artif Intern Organs. 1998;34:108–11.
97. Jenkins R, Harrison H, Chen B, et al. Accuracy of intravenous infusion pumps in continuous renal replacement therapies. Trans Am Soc Artif Intern Organs J. 1992;38:808–10.

98. McBryde KD, Bunchman TE, Kudelka TL, et al. Hyperosmolar solutions in continuous renal replacement therapy for hyperosmolar acute renal failure: a preliminary report. Pediatr Crit Care Med. 2005;6(2):228–39.
99. Barenbrock M, Hausberg M, Marzkies F, et al. Effects of bicarbonate- and lactate- buffered replacement fluids on cardiovascular outcome in CVVH patients. Kidney Int. 2000;58:1751–7.
100. Sethi SK, Bunchman TE, Raina R, Kher V. Unique considerations in renal replacement therapy in children: core curriculum 2014. Am J Kidney Dis. 2014;63:329–45.
101. Bunchman TE, Maxvold NJ, Barnett J, et al. Pediatric hemofiltration: Normocarb® dialysate solution with citrate anticoagulation. Pediatr Nephrol. 2002;17:150–4.
102. Levraut J, Ciebiera JP, Jambou P, et al. Effect of continuous venovenous hemofiltration with dialysis on lactate clearance in critically ill patients. Crit Care Med. 1997;25:58–62.
103. Cimochowski GE, Worley E, Rutherford WE, et al. Superiority of the internal jugular over the subclavian access for temporary dialysis. Nephron. 1990;54:154–61.

Chapter 4
CRRT Prescription

CRRT Technical Considerations

The CRRT prescription requires the selection of a properly functioning vascular access, appropriate catheter size, and low extracorporeal line sets and hemofilter as well as the purpose of treatment and availability of work team including experienced nursing staff, dietitian, pharmacist, and technical support. If one were to suggest a standard prescription, then a blood flow rate (BFR) for CVVH would be in the range of 4–6 mL/kg/min trying to keep a venous return pressure of less than 200 mmHg [1–7]. Further there is no absolute data to date on the rate of replacement fluid or dialysate fluid. Traditionally, we have used a rate of 2000 mL/1.73 m^2/h for this which allows us to compare pediatric data based on body surface area to adult data [1–7]. Thus, in a 10-kg child with a 0.5-m^2 body surface area, the dialysate or replacement fluid rate prescribed would be roughly 700 mL/h.

Factors affecting hemodynamics include excessive ultrafiltration and inadequate replacement. Vasopressor agents including epinephrine, norepinephrine, and dobutamine all have in common small molecular weight and minimal protein binding and are rapidly removed by plasma clearance.

Ultrafiltration Rates (Removal Rates)

Each dialyzer has a specified ultrafiltration coefficient that is a measure of fluid that will pass from the membrane in 1 h. Dividing the fluid removal desired by hours of treatment gives the ultrafiltration rate. The amount ultrafiltered depends on transmembrane pressure between the blood and dialysate compartment.

F. Assadi, F.G. Sharbaf, *Pediatric Continuous Renal Replacement Therapy*,
DOI 10.1007/978-3-319-26202-4_4

The rate of ultrafiltration depends on the patient's hemodynamic status. In children, a dose ranging from 35 to 40 mL/kg/h or 2 to 3 L/1.73 m^2 of either connective or diffusive clearance would provide adequate urea clearance [1, 4, 8]. It is recommended to start ultrafiltration with zero and slowly increase to 1–2 mL/kg/h or 0.5–3 L/1.73 m^2/h until fluid balance goal is achieved [1, 4, 5, 8].

Calculating the Desired Patient Fluid Removal Rate

The CRRT machine software automatically calculates the ultrafiltration rate needed to achieve the patient fluid removal rate (FRR). The machine "control unit software," however, does not measure or account for non-CRRT sources of patient fluid intake (such as hyperalimentation and blood or drug infusion) or fluid output (such as urine and wound drainage). It also does not account for anticoagulant solution infused for CRRT modality anticoagulant syringe pump. The operator must account for those sources when calculating the patient FRR, as well as when calculating the patient's input/output totals.

Blood Flow Rates

A minimum of 30–50 mL/min blood flow is required to minimize access and filter clotting. The maximum BFR is 400 mL/min/1.73 m^2 or 10–12 mL/kg/min in neonates and infants, 4–6 mL/kg/min in children, and 2–4 mL/kg/min in adolescents (Table 4.1).

The BFR generated by the PRISMA machine ranges from 5 to 10 mL/kg/min (up to 180 mL/min), which will allow adequate flow through the circuit [1, 4, 5, 8]. We use a minimum of 50 mL/min for newborn infants. The venous pressure should be preferably no higher than 250 mmHg. Table 4.1 demonstrates the recommended BFR during CRRT for pediatric patients.

Dialysate/Replacement Solution Flow Rates

The ultrafiltration rate/plasma flow rate (BFR × (1-Hct) ratio should be <0.35–0.4 in order to avoid filter clotting. Dialysate or effluent flow rates ranging from 20 to 35 mL/min/m^2 (~2000 mL/h/1.73 m^2) are usually adequate (adult data). The standard dialysate flow rate is 40–60 mL/kg/h or 2.5 L/h/1.73 m^2 [1, 4, 8].

Table 4.1 Choosing blood flow rate for pediatric CRRT

Body weight (kg)	<10	11–20	21–50 kg	>50
Blood flow rate (mL/min)	24–50	80–100	100–150	150–180

All CRRT techniques other than SCUF require the use of dialysate or replacement solution to compensate for the effluent fluid and electrolyte removal. Optimal dialysate or replacement solution approximates normal plasma water composition, replacing electrolytes and minerals in physiologic concentrations without replacing the metabolic solutes, which accumulate in AKI. The composition of these solutions can be varied extensively to achieve specific metabolic goals (e.g., bicarbonate-based solutions can be used to correct acidemia and the electrolyte content can be altered to correct electrolyte imbalance) [8–14].

When citrate anticoagulation is used in CRRT, modifications are necessary in both the replacement fluid and dialysate [15–19]. Citrate is metabolized to bicarbonate by the liver; therefore, buffer is not generally required in the dialysate [9, 20–26]. Similarly, dialysate used in citrate regional anticoagulation is generally hyponatremic to prevent hypernatremia, and it is recommended that fluids are calcium-free. Few commercially available calcium-free, bicarbonate-based CRRT fluids have been available until recently.

Lactate- and acetate-based solutions are no longer recommended for patients with multiorgan failure undergoing CRRT because of patients' limited capacity to convert these buffers to bicarbonate [11, 27].

Bicarbonate-based solutions are the solution of choice for patients under CRRT [14]. Patients on CRRT tend to develop hypophosphatemia. However, a combination of bicarbonate, calcium, and phosphorus in the same bag may increase the risk of precipitation. To avoid this, phosphorus should be given to the patient in a line separate from the circuit. The bicarbonate concentration in the solution should be lowered to 22–25 mEq/L to avoid metabolic alkalosis, if a citrate anticoagulation protocol is used.

There is no absolute data to date on the rate of replacement fluid or dialysate fluid. A rate of 2 L/h/1.73 m^2 is recommended for pediatrics CRRT (CVVH, CVVHD, CVVHDF).

Net Fluid Balance

Fluid balance should take into account the patient's hemodynamics status, volume status, and fluid requirements. A suggested net ultrafiltration per hour is 2 L/1.73 m^2/h [1, 4, 8]. Aggressive ultrafiltration should be avoided in hemodynamic unstable patients. In such setting, solute clearance can be achieved without ultrafiltration.

The system is very efficient; thus, too much fluid can be removed too quickly. This is the perfect time to maximize the total parenteral nutrition (TPN) of the patient. Further, in order to get maximum fluid shift with colloid infusion, the ultrafiltration rate for the colloid previously infused should be over twice as much as the colloid rate "in" (e.g., 200 mL of PRBCs infused over 2 h should be ultrafiltrated over 4 h).

The patient net FRR that should be set on the CRRT machine control unit may be calculated using the following formula:

$$\begin{aligned}&\text{Patient FRR}\left(\text{mL}/\text{h}\right)\\&\text{set in CRRT machine}=\left[\text{Net fluid removal}\left(\text{UD}\right)\text{rate}\left(\text{mL}/\text{h}\right)+\text{fluid intake}\right.\\&\qquad\left.\left(\text{IV, TPN, citrate, calcium infusion rates}\left(\text{mL}/\text{h}\right)\right)\right]\\&\qquad-\left[\text{Non-CRRT 0.5em outputs}\left(\text{mL}/\text{h}\right)\text{urine, 0.5em etc.}\right]\end{aligned}$$

The patient net FRR must be adjusted if the weight loss prescribed by the physician is changed or if the patient's non-PRISMA fluid inputs or outputs change.

Circuit Priming

Priming a hemofilter circuit is recommended when circuit volume is >10 % of patient's intravascular blood volume. Heparinized 0.9 % saline (5000 U/L) is commonly used for most patients. Smaller patients require blood priming to prevent hypotension particularly when the circuit volume is >10–15 % patient blood volume.

Risks of using blood for prime include bradykinin release syndrome (bronchospasm, hypotension, mucosal congestion), hyperkalemia, hyponatremia, and hypocalcemia [28, 29]. The pH of blood coming in contact with electronegatively charged membranes during prime elicits bradykinin response especially in patients <10 kg (standard blood from a blood bank has a pH of 6.4). The lower the pH, the more bradykinin released from blood. Saline (pH 5.0) does not elicit a bradykinin response because it does not contain bradykinin or other blood substances. CRRT membrane AN-69 is highly biocompatible with low thrombogenicity and electronegative surface. Its use has been associated with a bradykinin release syndrome particularly in patients on ACE inhibitors or in acidotic patients. Blood-banked blood has a pH of 6.4 with calcium being essentially zero. This has been shown to cause the bradykinin release syndrome that clinically appears to be anaphylaxis associated with acute hypotension, tachycardia, and a drop in the CVP. This is immediately reversible by removing the system and may be avoided by buffering the blood or by post-hemofiltration blood transfusion [28, 29].

The blood buffer solution can be prepared by mixing 43 mL of blood-banked blood with 7 mL of THAM, 50 mL of a solution of 150 mEq of $NaHCO_3$ in 1000 mL of water, 45 mg of $CaCl_2$, and 2 U/mL of heparin. The final pH of this is 7.41 and the Ca^{++} is 1.0 mmol/L. 90 mL of this combination may be used for blood priming and may prevent bradykinin release syndrome. Following blood transfusion, monitor the child's pH and give sufficient $NaHCO_3$ to the child to bring the pH to > 7.35.

Anticoagulation

Many children who require CRRT will need anticoagulation to prevent filter membrane clotting and blood loss [15–19, 30]. Insufficient anticoagulation may affect filter longevity and decreases dialyzer efficiency and performance. On the other hand, excessive anticoagulation may result in bleeding complications or thrombocytopenia [31–35]. The adult data on the use of regional citrate anticoagulation during CRRT show a decreased risk of bleeding and at the least equivalent circuit survival as compared to heparin. Current pediatric and adult studies support regional citrate anticoagulation as an effective alternative to systemic heparin anticoagulation in most patient populations.

Heparin-Free CRRT

CRRT can be performed without anticoagulation, especially in children with high risk of bleeding. Children with activated clotting time (ACT) >200 s, low platelet count, and liver failure can also be treated without the use of anticoagulation [33, 35].

Multiple organ dysfunction syndrome classically occurs in patients who also suffer from abnormal clotting parameters. Usually these patients are given ample amount of platelet infusions and coagulation factors. This excessive amount of volume adds to greater need for ultrafiltration and greater risk for clotting.

In heparin-free CRRT, blood flows are maintained above 5–10 mL/min, and saline flushes should be administered (40–45 mL) every 15–30 min into the arterial limb of the circuit to maintain circuit patency.

Heparin Protocol

Systemic administration of heparin with protamine infusion back to the patient should be avoided because it does not improve circuit life and may cause coagulopathy in the patient [15–19, 30]. Heparin is generally administered as a bolus (10–20 U/kg), followed by continuous infusion (10–20 U/kg/h) into the arterial limb of the CRRT circuit (pre-filter) to maintain ACT between 180 and 200 s or partial thromboplastin time of two times normal. The infusion rate of heparin is adjusted to the keep the ACT at target level between 170 and 220 s (Table 4.2). ACT should be checked every 1–4 h on the "venous" side of the hemofilter, meaning after the hemofilter (post-filter). Adjust post-filter ACT between 180 and 200 s. If ACT is

Table 4.2 Heparin dosing adjustment during CRRT[a]

If the ACT is	Make this change
170–220	No change
>220	HOLD heparin for 1 h, then decrease the infusion by 10 % less/hour, and recheck ACT in an hour
<170	Administer bolus of 10 U/kg, then increase the infusion by 10 %, and recheck ACT in an hour

[a]References [15–19, 30]

>150 or <180 s, then no load is necessary; just start the drip. If ACT is >200, no heparin is necessary and recheck in 30 min for 2–3 h. Once an established ACT pattern is identified, then check ACT q4 h (Table 4.2).

Heparin Dose Adjustment

Determine heparin concentration as follows:

Patient weight	Heparin concentration[a] (U/mL)
<10 kg	40
11–25 kg	100
16–60 kg	250
>60 kg	500

[a]PRISMA heparin rate must be ≥0.5 mL/h

Initial bolus is 20 U/kg (administer pre-filter). Subsequent hourly continuous infusion (10–20 U/kg/h) is given to maintain APTT of 1.5–2.5 times the control value (25–35 s).

Adjust heparin infusion rate according to APTT as follows:

APTT (s)	Heparin infusion rate
50–80	No change
<50	Administer bolus of 10 U/kg, increase by 10 %, and recheck APPT in 1 h
>80	Hold heparin infusion by ½ h, decrease by 10 %, and recheck APPT in 1 h

Patients who develop heparin-induced thrombocytopenia (HIT) frequently need further anticoagulation to treat an ongoing thromboembolic problem or to prevent one. Orgaran, a low-molecular-weight (LMW) glycosaminoglycuronan, has shown a low frequency (10 %) of cross-reactivity in vitro with sera containing the HIT antibody, in contrast to the much higher frequency of cross-reactivity (approximately 80 %) shown by the LMW heparins [33, 35]. This study summarizes the results of intravenous or subcutaneous Orgaran treatment in 57 patients, in whom the diagnosis of HIT was reasonably confirmed by exclusion of other causes of thrombocytopenia and by objective tests. The presenting indications for Orgaran were continuous veno-venous hemofiltration and hemodialysis ($n=21$), thromboembolism treatment ($n=23$), thromboembolism prophylaxis ($n=10$), and anticoagulation for coronary artery bypass graft ($n=4$), peripheral bypass graft surgery, and plasmapheresis ($n=1$ each). The results showed Orgaran to be a safe, well-tolerated, effective (successful treatment in over 90 % of patients) anticoagulant in patients with a high thrombotic and/or bleeding risk even if critically ill and requiring hemofiltration.

Low-molecular-weight heparin has higher anti-x and is a more reliable anticoagulant than heparin. Its pharmacokinetics is more predictable because of less plasma protein binding. However, there are no significant differences between the low-molecular-weight heparin and unfractionated heparin in reduced risk of bleeding, thrombocytopenia, or filter life. Low-molecular-weight heparin will accumulate in patients with AKI and should not be used in patients with AKI, as the drug will accumulate during CRRT. If used, follow anti-factor Xa levels and reduce the dosing interval.

Citrate Dextrose (ACD)

Clotting is a calcium-dependent mechanism. Removal of calcium from the blood will inhibit clotting. Adding citrate to blood will bind the ionized calcium in the blood thus inhibiting clotting. The use of citrate anticoagulation has become increasingly popular [10, 18, 20–22, 24–26, 34, 36–39]. Unlike heparin, citrate has no effect upon patient bleeding, and it is easy to administer and monitor with calcium assay and is cost effective. Regional citrate anticoagulation is performed using a continuous infusion through the arterial limb of the circuit. The citrate chelates free Ca^{++} and the citrate-calcium complex is removed by CRRT, which inhibits the coagulation cascade. Therefore, plasma Ca^{++} levels should be maintained with the use of a continuous Ca^{++} infusion.

Citrate anticoagulation requires a separate central line (for calcium infusion). The infusion rate of citrate is adjusted to maintain target blood ACT level (Table 4.3). Regional citrate infusion requires the use of a commercially available solution and frequent monitoring of plasma Ca^{++} level (Table 4.4).

Citrate Protocol for CVVH (PRISMA)

1. Prime tin CVVHDF mode using dialysate (bicarbonate based without calcium) and replacement solutions.
2. Obtain from pharmacy 1000 mL anticoagulant citrate dextrose (ACD) solution and connect the ACD to a regular iv pump and attach it to the "pre-hemofilter arterial" 3-way stopcock.
3. Infuse ACD rate (mL/min) at 1.5 × BFR (mL/min) (for instance, if PRISMA BFR is 100 mL/min, start ACD at 150 mL/h).
4. In children less than 10 kg who are receiving blood transfusion, avoid the use of ACD for the first 15 min to prevent or retard the bradykinin release syndrome seen in some patients.
5. Start the calcium chloride infusion (8 g in 1 L 0.9 % saline) at 40 % of the ACD flow rate via the central line other than the dialysis access (for instance, if the

Table 4.3 Anticoagulation protocol[a]

❑ Heparin ------------- U/ml in 20mL syringe
Deliver on heparin syringe line
Loading dose: (20U/kg)_________
Continuous infusion rate (5-20U/kg)____U/kg/h

ACT	Heparin adjustment
<170	10-20U/kg bolus and Increase dose by 10% and recheck ACT 1h
170-220	No change
>220	Hold heparin for 1h, then restart at 10% reduced dose and recheck ACT 1h

❑ *Citrate (ACD-A)
Starting rate: 1.5 X BFR_______mL/h
Must use systemic on the pre-filter of the hemofiltration access

Post-filter ionized calcium (mmol/L)	Citrate adjustment
<0.25	Decrease by 5 mL/h
0.25-0.39	No change
0.40-0.50	Increase by 5 mL/h
>0.5	Increase by 10 mL/h

* Must order calcium chloride infusion

❑ *Calcium Chloride:
8.0 g in 1000 ml 0.9% saline
Starting rate: 0.4 X ACD-A______ mL/h
Deliver via IV pump on return line

Systemic ionized calcium (mmol/L)	Calcium chloride adjustment
>1.3	Decrease by 10mL/h
1.1-1.3	No change
0.9-1.1	Increase by 10 mL/h
<0.9	Increase by 20 mL/h
<0.9 or > 1.3	Call Nephrologist

* Must order citrate infusion

[a]**References [10, 15–22, 24–26, 30, 34, 36–40]**

Table 4.4 Titrate the calcium infusion according to the calcium sliding scale

Patient ionized Ca^{++} (mmol/L)	Calcium infusion adjustment	
	>20 kg	<20 kg
>1.3	↓ rate by 10 mL/h	↓ rate by 5 mL/h
1.1–1.3 (optimum range)	No adjustment	
0.9–1.1	↑ rate by 10 mL/h	↑ rate by 5 mL/h
<0.9	↑ rate by 20 mL/h	↑ rate by 10 mL/h

Notify MD if calcium infusion rate >200 mL/h

citrate rate is 150 mL/h, then the calcium chloride rate will be 60 mL/h) (Tables 4.4 and 4.5).

6. Set flow rates in PRIMA as ordered.
7. Calculate patient FRR by using the following equation:

$$\text{FRR} = \text{Net ultrafiltration rate} + \text{ACD rate} + \text{Calcium infusion rate}$$

8. Connect the CVVH (PRISMA circuit) to the dialysis catheter and press the start key.
9. Draw blood 2 h after initiation of ACD infusion and every 6 h thereafter for post-hemofilter (the return line) for ionized calcium and from peripheral blood or from patient arterial line for electrolytes, BUN, creatinine, ionized calcium, phosphorus, and albumin.
10. Titrate the ACD infusion according to the citrate sliding scale (Table 4.4).
11. Titrate the calcium infusion according to the calcium sliding scale (Table 4.5).
12. If serum bicarbonate falls below 35 mEq/L, add 0.9 % saline (200–400 mL/h) as replacement solution and decrease the dialysate rate by the same amount. This will give an acid load from the normal saline and lowers the bicarbonate from the bath at the same time.
13. If the patient systemic blood ionized calcium falls below 0.75 mmol/L, stop ACD infusion for 1 h and resume infusion at 30 % of citrate flow rate. Also administer bolus of 10 mg/kg of calcium chloride and increase calcium infusion by 10 %.
14. If the serum sodium is greater than 150 mEq/L, change replacement fluid to 0.45 % saline.
15. If the filter clots, stop the ACD and calcium infusions and replace the filter.

Citrate is metabolized to bicarbonate by the liver; as a result, buffer is not generally required in the dialysate.

Citrate infusion is recommended in patients targeted for heparin-free CRRT and those requiring lower BFR. Filter life above 96 h is common with citrate anticoagulation and it does not cause HIT syndrome.

The disadvantages of using citrate anticoagulation include hypocalcemia, hypomagnesemia, hypernatremia, metabolic alkalosis, and citrate toxicity in patients with liver failure.

Table 4.5 Anticoagulant agents for CRRT[a]

Anticoagulant agent	Filter prime	Initial dose	Maintenance dose	Monitoring	Comments
0.9 % saline solution	2 L saline	150–250 mL pre-filter	100–250 mL/h pre-filter	Visual check	No anticoagulant used
Heparin	2500–10,000 U/2 L saline	5–10 U/kg	3–12 U/kg/h	ACT 200–250; PTT 1.5–2.0 × normal	Simple and easy to use
LMW heparin	2 L saline	40 mg	10–40 mg/6 h	Factor Xa levels; maintained between 0.1 and 0.41 U/mL	Lower risk of bleeding
Regional heparin	2500 U/2 L saline	5–10 U/kg	31–12 U/kg/h; +protamine post-filter	PTT: post-filter ACT 200–250	Lower risk of bleeding
Regional citrate	2 L saline	4 % trisodium citrate 150–180 mL/h	100–180 mL/h 3–7 % of BFR, Ca replaced by central line 4–8 ng/kg/min	ACT: 200–250; maintain ionized calcium 1.0–1.2 nmol/L	No bleeding; no thrombocytopenia; better filter efficacy, longevity

[a]References [10, 15–22, 24–26, 30, 34, 36–40]

In children who receive "blood priming" and are on citrate anticoagulation, withhold the citrate for the first 10–15 min until hemodynamic stability is achieved. During this time, if needed, give 20 U/kg of heparin as one-time dose to anticoagulate the system until the citrate is begun. Citrate is acidic and may exacerbate the bradykinin release reaction.

The combination of bicarbonate-based solutions with bicarbonate concentrations >30 mEq/L and citrate anticoagulation often will result in metabolic alkalosis. Therefore, if citrate anticoagulation is used, it is preferred to use a replacement solution with bicarbonate level between 22 and 25 mEq/L as well as a zero calcium bath.

In summary, regional citrate anticoagulation is gaining popularity for CRRT in the critically ill patient, with either similar or longer CRRT circuit life compared to standard systemic anticoagulation with unfractionated or LMW heparins, but with reduced risk of hemorrhage and blood transfusion requirement. The dose of citrate needs to adjusted for blood flow, to achieve a pre-hemofilter/dialyzer ionized calcium target of <0.25 mmol/L, approximately corresponding to a citrate concentration of 4–6 mmol/L, for effective anticoagulation. Calcium is then reinfused to maintain a normal systemic ionized calcium concentration, and the citrate infusion adjusted according to the post-filter ionized calcium and the total systemic serum calcium. Patients can become alkalotic due to the metabolism of an increasing citrate load returning to the patient but also acidotic if citrate cannot be readily metabolized or the amount of citrate infused is too low. In addition, this may be compounded by nursing and/or fluid composition errors. However, by carefully monitoring ionized and total calcium, appropriate adjustments can be made to dialysate and/or replacement fluid rates and citrate and/or calcium infusion rates, to achieve acid–base targets. Although citrate is predominantly metabolized by the liver, many patients with liver disease, even those with cirrhosis, can often adequately metabolize the citrate load.

Prostacyclin

Prostacyclin (epoprostenol), a potent vasodilator and antithrombotic and antiplatelet agent, has been safely used to prevent clotting of the extracorporeal circuits either alone in patients with thrombocytopenia and/or increased risk of bleeding or in combination with heparin in a state of hypercoagulability [41].

Prostacyclin infusion pre-filter decreases bleeding risk without increasing platelet consumption. Systemic administration of prostacyclin does not prolong filter life during CVVH (www.pcrrt.com). Initial dose is 4 ng/kg/min (range 2–8 ng/kg/min). Monitor circuit life. If less than 48 h, increase sequentially by 2 ng/kg/min to max of 8 ng/kg/min. Closely monitor side effects (hypotension, facial flushing, hyperthermia, headache).

Nutrition

Adequate feeding of critically ill patients under continuous renal replacement therapy (CRRT) remains a challenging issue. AKI increases catabolic state and alters amino acid metabolism leading to high level of urea nitrogen production.

CRRT allows clearance of LMW water-soluble substances including significant loss of glucose, amino acids, LMW proteins, trace elements, water-soluble vitamins, small peptides, and electrolytes [23, 42–47]. The range of amino acid and protein losses on CRRT is estimated to be between 1.2 and 7 g/day. Amino acid and protein losses represent between 10 and 12 % of total delivered nutritional proteins. Glutamine loss accounts for approximately 20 % of total amino acid loss. If not recognized and corrected in time, depletion of specific substances will become harmful for the patient.

Malnutrition remains one of the most troublesome complications of AKI and should be managed as a collaborative venture with dietitians, pharmacists, and nursing staff. Malnutrition is usually multifactorial in origin and may reflect anorexia, restricted diet, the catabolic nature of the underlying disease (e.g., sepsis, rhabdomyolysis), nutrient losses in drainage fluid or dialysate, and reduced synthesis of muscle protein [23, 42–47].

Calories

The aim of dietary therapy in AKI is to provide sufficient calories (100–110 kcal/kg/day) to avoid catabolism and starvation ketoacidosis, while minimizing production of nitrogenous waste. This is best achieved by restricting dietary protein to approximately 1.0 g/kg/day of protein of high biological value and by providing calories in the form of carbohydrates. Higher protein intake is recommended in catabolic patients or those with a prolonged maintenance phase, even if it precipitates the need for dialysis. Indeed, management of nutrition is easier after institution of dialysis when patients are generally prescribed 1.5–2.0 g protein/kg/day. Vigorous parenteral hyperalimentation has been claimed to improve prognosis in AKI patients receiving CRRT [23, 42–47].

Recommended daily energy and protein requirements during CRRT range from 25 to 35 kcal/kg (with proportionally 60–70 % carbohydrates and 30–40 % lipids) and from 1.5 to 1.8 g/kg body weight, respectively.

Glucose

Glucose loss can be estimated by multiplying the glucose concentration measured in an aliquot of effluent with the total daily effluent volume. However, adding glucose to CRRT solutions may be problematic and CRRT mass transfer dynamics for glucose are insufficiently clarified. Supplementing glucose to the replacement fluid may produce a net glucose uptake as high as 300 g/day in patients under CRRT. This amount of glucose is the highest permitted to obviate hepatic lipid accumulation, which disturbs liver metabolism. When glucose is added to the substitution fluid, a progressive increase in glucose concentration is noted with linear increments in net glucose transfer to the patient. Whether glucose-enriched solutions eventually affect ultrafiltration capacity and dose delivery during high-flux hemodiafiltration with polysulfone membranes is poorly studied. Finally, both higher plasma glucose levels and a higher glucose turnover have been described when lactate-based solutions are employed. Although it remains unclear if glucose losses should be compensated, current evidence suggests that keeping glycemia within the normal range is beneficial. Most routinely used substitution fluids do contain dextrose and strict glycemia control during CRRT is thus essential. Continuous glucose monitoring in patients on extracorporeal treatment, including CRRT, may be the best option to anticipate for dysglycemia problems [23, 42–47].

Proteins

CRRT produces a significant nitrogen loss, which if not properly supplemented, may result in a negative nitrogen balance. Amino acids have different rates of elimination during extended CRRT, and losses need to be counterbalanced by increasing the protein supply by approximately 3–4 g/kg/day to assure a positive nitrogen balance in these highly catabolic patients. Since nutritional support is not volume limited during CRRT, adequate amounts of protein can be provided to compensate for losses [23, 42–47].

Lipids

AKI is associated with increased triglyceride content of low-density lipoproteins, altered lipolysis, and reduced hepatic lipase activity. Taken together, this impaired lipid metabolism may cause an up to 50 % decrease of lipid, and especially triglyceride, clearance. This enhances the risk of hyperglycemia particularly in parenterally fed patients. Due to lower breakdown, triglycerides accumulate in AKI patients. Triglyceride overload becomes problematic when parenteral nutrition is started and is not resolved by CRRT because the very high molecular weight of these substances precludes filtration. Thus, triglyceride levels need close monitoring in patients with AKI treated by CRRT especially when receiving parenteral nutrition. Both high molecular weight and inherent lack of water solubility preclude lipid elimination by CRRT. Lipids may also become involved in early packing or clotting of filters when unfractionated heparin is used as anticoagulant. This is seen less with citrate [23, 42–47].

Vitamins and Trace Elements

Patients with AKI receiving CRRT are prone to depletion of trace elements. Reasons are multifactorial and include variable protein binding, redistribution between plasma and tissues, acute loss of biological fluids, dilution, varying concentrations of trace elements in dialysis/hemofiltration fluids, nutrient intake, and removal from plasma by CRRT. Water-soluble vitamin and trace element losses and requirements during CRRT remain the subject of debate and research. In general, water-soluble vitamins are highly removed by CRRT. Proposed recommendations for daily supplementation of water-soluble vitamins are 100 mg vitamin B1, 2 mg vitamin B2, 20 mg vitamin B3, 10 mg vitamin B5, 200 mg biotin, 1 mg folic acid, 4 μg vitamin B12, and 250 mg vitamin C. Thiamine loss may largely exceed the daily provision of this vitamin by standard TPN. Therefore, recommended supplements may vary accordingly.

The fat-soluble vitamins E and K also need to be supplemented (10 IU/day and 4 mg/week respectively), but vitamin A must be reduced to compensate for deficient retinol degradation. Daily parenteral supplementation with standard doses of trace elements is supposed to compensate for CRRT removal. However, the optimal dose of trace element preparations in patients on CRRT is currently unknown. Trace element losses are most often intercepted by tripling the dose of currently available intravenous trace element-containing solutions, even in enterally fed patients. Among the trace elements, selenium may become significantly depleted during CRRT. Therefore, an additional intravenous dose of 100 μg (at least 20–60 μg) selenium should be administered daily during CRRT. To date, supplementation of vitamins and trace elements during CRRT has shown no proven benefit on survival [23, 42–47].

Electrolytes

Hypokalemia is present in 5–25 % of patients treated with CRRT and is mainly due to inadequate potassium supplementation. Paradoxically, potassium loss is easily avoided either by using potassium-rich replacement fluids in hemofiltration, altering potassium concentration in the substitution fluid, or administration of potassium supplements. Serum potassium levels below 3 mEq/L should absolutely be avoided as rapid correction may increase mortality. Clinicians typically tend to avoid hyperkalemia in patients on CRRT [48]. However, if hypervolemia is the main indication for initiating CRRT, hyperkalemia usually is innocuous and potassium substitution within the normal blood concentration range should be encouraged. Low potassium-containing fluids are only mandatory in markedly life-threatening hyperkalemia.

Further, in phosphorus-deficient dialysate solutions (none have phosphorus unless added by a local pharmacy), hypophosphatemia occurs frequently, requiring either a separate phosphorus infusion or additional phosphorus added to the TPN.

The incidence of hypophosphatemia during CRRT varies between 10.9 and 65 %. Its clinical effect remains poorly defined, yet phosphorus is involved in many vital functions such as tissue support, enzymatic processes, oxygen transport, and energy transfer. Hypophosphatemia has been associated with failure to wean from mechanical ventilation in medical ICU patients. Adding phosphorus to substitution fluids is safe and adequately compensates undesired losses. Commercial fluids containing physiological phosphate concentrations are to be preferred because they permit minimalization of the contamination risk and avoidance of eventual dosing errors when using “homemade” solutions. To compensate phosphorus loss, either intravenous bolus or enteral supplements can be administered. Special emphasis should be given whenever refeeding syndrome is suspected. Recommendations do suggest that phosphate levels should be controlled at least twice daily during CRRT [23, 42–47, 49].

Hyperphosphatemia rarely occurs during CRRT and, if present, requires increased clearance and the use of phosphate-free dialysis fluids. Phosphate is largely located intracellularly. Thus, a persistently high phosphorus level during CRRT may be a marker of massive intracellular necrosis (e.g., severe bowel ischemia). Hypomagnesemia is rarely seen (<3 %) and easily corrected with either commercially available fluids or daily administration of 2–4 g intravenous magnesium salt boluses. Regarding calcium, hypocalcemia is commonly reported as a side effect with an incidence of up to 50 % in some case series. With the rising use of diluted citrate, calcium is more easily corrected as compared to the heparin era. It has also been shown that hypercalcemia can be more easily controlled by CRRT and especially by avoiding rebound hypercalcemia.

Consensus exists to supplement important micronutrients such as amino acids (glutamine), water-soluble vitamins, and trace elements. Critically ill patients with AKI on CRRT can lose 15–30 % of amino acids. They also can lose significant vitamins and minerals during CRRT. In patients on CRRT, in order to maintain adequate nitrogen balance, protein administration should be in the range of 3–4 g/kg/day. In phosphorus-deficient dialysate solutions, hypophosphatemia occurs frequently, requiring either a separate phosphorus infusion or additional phosphorus added to a nutritional supplement [23, 42–47, 49, 50].

CRRT Complications and Troubleshootings

CRRT is an accepted therapy for the management of renal insufficiency or renal failure in critically ill patients from neonates to adults. The therapy is more technologically challenging in small infants and children due to the size of the vessels, which mandates the use of smaller catheters [51–53]. Knowledge of the systems used, potential complications, and alarm troubleshooting make the therapy feasible despite these challenges.

CRRT-related complications are potentially serious [28, 48, 54–56]. The most common are hypotension at the time of connection and electrolyte disturbances [29, 56, 57]. Strict control and continuous monitoring of the technique are therefore necessary in children on CRRT.

Vascular Access Spasm

Complications of vascular access, including infection and vascular injury, are a common concern with continuous renal replacement therapy. These complications are reported to occur in 5–19 % of patients, depending on the access site selected.

Arterial puncture, hematoma, hemothorax, and pneumothorax are the most common complications reported. Arteriovenous fistulas, aneurysms, thrombus formation, and retroperitoneal hemorrhage have also been described.

Vascular spasm is usually due to the high initial BFR, movement of catheter against the vessel wall, or improper length of hemodialysis catheter inserted.

While current systems generally are used to provide veno-venous hemofiltration, the term arterial often is used to describe the blood removal or access side of the system. Venous describes the return side of the system.

Low arterial pressure alarms indicate a problem with troubleshooting mechanical complications in CRRT pulling blood from the patient's catheter. This may be the result of a physical obstruction such as a clamp left in place, a kink in the catheter or tubing, or a clot in that portion of the system. It also may indicate that the pump speed is too fast for the size of the catheter, causing the catheter to pull against the side of the vessel and resulting in obstruction to outflow. In the pediatric patient, this also can occur when the pump speed is too fast for the central venous pressure or amount of blood available in the right atrium.

Venous pressure alarms indicate a problem with blood returning to the patient. High venous pressure results from an obstruction to blood return. Again, this can be the result of a clamp left engaged on the return side, a kink in the catheter or tubing, or a clot in the venous return system. Conversely, a low venous pressure alarm may occur when the system does not sense venous flow or positive pressure on the return limb of the circuit. This can result from a disconnection on the venous side of the system, from obstruction between the filter and venous pressure sensor, or from a pump speed too low to produce positive pressure in a larger venous catheter.

Transmembrane pressure alarms indicate a change in the pressure across the membrane, between the blood and ultrafiltrate compartments. This is usually indicative of a failing filter. As the filter ages, micro-clotting occurs within the fibers, decreasing the area for filtration, thus increasing the transmembrane pressure to achieve the same ultrafiltration rate. On some systems, this alarm also can occur if a clamp inadvertently is left in place on the ultrafiltrate tubing; other machines have a separate ultrafiltration alarm.

Excessive Ultrafiltration

Excessive ultrafiltration usually occurs when the intravenous pumps are used to regulate ultrafiltration. The only way to avoid this error is to use industry-made equipment that is highly recommended for ultrafiltration regulation [1, 40, 58–63].

Current systems used for CRRT have a variety of alarms that indicate changes or problems with the prescribed fluid balance. It is important to pay close attention to these, especially in the pediatric patient, as minimal changes in fluid balance can have significant patient consequences. One of these alarms is an ultrafiltration alarm indicating that the amount of ultrafiltration prescribed is not being met. Another is a balance or bag volume/weight alarm indicating that the amount of ultrafiltrate, replacement fluid, or dialysate is outside the prescribed volume. Each system has a small window/percentage of error to prevent the pump from sounding the alarm continuously. Once the weight or balance is outside this window, an alarm will sound. Typically, fluid balance alarms occur due to bags being clamped or the scales being moved after the pump is moved or secondary to other concurrent alarms.

Membrane Reactions

One of the more biocompatible membranes (PAN, AN-69) has been shown to cause a bradykinin release syndrome in patients who are acidotic at the onset of CRRT or in children who require a "blood prime" in the setting of one of these membranes [28, 29]. These membranes, in the face of interacting with an acidotic plasma environment, generate bradykinin, which may result in reactions from minor nausea to clinical anaphylaxis. Newer AN-69 membranes are now coming to the market that will prevent these reactions. In the meantime, in those patients who require blood priming, transfusing the blood post-hemofilter with a generous administration of sodium bicarbonate or the use of a priming mixture of 75 mL PRBC, 75 mL sodium bicarbonate, and 300 mg calcium gluconate makes this reaction virtually nonexistent. Alternate formulas exist for priming including "the Jenkins formula": pRBC = 80 mL; 5 % albumin = 55 mL; heparin = 150 U; sodium bicarbonate = 12 mEq; and 10 % calcium gluconate = 2 mL. The prime must then be checked to be sure that the pH is 7.3–7.5 and the ionized calcium is ≥1.0.

Hypothermia

CRRT is associated with a higher incidence of hypothermia. CRRT-induced body cooling is determined both by the time during which blood circulates outside the body and the contact with cold dialysate and/or replacement fluids. Long-term body cooling may have unwarranted or potentially detrimental side effects such as energy loss, shivering with increased oxygen demand, vasoconstriction, impairment of leukocyte function, and coagulation disorders. As a consequence, monitoring of body temperature is imperative. If the incorporated CRRT heating system fails to maintain the desired core temperature, external heating aiming at a temperature above 37 °C (and sometimes even close to 42 °C) must be utilized. Of note, cooling may beneficially affect hemodynamics and outcome in ICU patients. As such, CRRT has proven useful to quickly establish hypothermia in certain conditions (e.g., cardiac arrest induced by ventricular fibrillation).

CRRT provokes a heat loss of approximately 1000 kcal/day, which must be considered into the energy balance account. On the contrary, and especially during shock, overzealous hypothermia may be deleterious for myocardial function and should be carefully monitored especially also regarding clotting and platelet count. Ideally, energy requirements should be measured by indirect calorimetry to more correctly match the amount of delivered calories to the patient's needs. Indirect calorimetry, however, remains difficult to perform during CRRT because the CRRT-induced bicarbonate/CO_2 diversion renders the measurement unreliable. At room temperature, CRRT produces loads of CO_2. This production will increase during active rewarming of the substitution fluid or the blood itself. In other words, during CRRT, CO_2 production no longer reflects the metabolic production of the body because substantial amounts of CO_2 are produced by the transformation of bicarbonate during CRRT. To overcome this inconvenience, indirect calorimetry could be performed when the patient is off CRRT. Currently, we conduct a randomized crossover study comparing indirect calorimetry in patients on and off CRRT, using patients within one study group as their own controls. The major aim is to quantify the bicarbonate/CO_2 diversion and to determine a factor for correcting indirect calorimetry results during CRRT. More generally speaking, dose is by far the most important item that may interfere with nutrition needs. Intermittent hemodialysis does obviously need completely different guidelines.

Although hypothermia is common, however, with the advent of thermic controllers, this has become less of a clinical problem. In the smaller child on hemofilter, a thermic controller will result in euthermia but may mask a fever; therefore, a high index of suspicion of new or ongoing infection needs to be maintained even in the absence of a fever. Techniques for thermic control include circuit warming blankets and dialysate/replacement fluid warmer. A blood warmer should be placed on the return line closest to the access. Monitor closely the patient's body temperature during CRRT.

Patients who do not require warming interventions are most likely febrile.

Infections

Infection is the most serious complication of AKI, occurs in about 50–90 % of cases, and accounts for as many as 70 % of deaths [64].

Bleeding

Anemia and thrombocytopenia may require transfusion in patients with symptoms or with active bleeding [32]. Unless there is active blood loss (e.g., bleeding, hemolysis), a good rule of thumb is that in a child <10 kg, 3.5 cc/kg will increase the Hct by 3 %, while in a child >10 kg, 3 cc/kg of PRBCs will increase a child's Hct by 3 %.

Circuit Clotting

The complications associated with CRRT in children are predominately related to spasm due to high blood flow, movement of catheter against vascular wall, improper length of catheter inserted, bleeding, infections, clotting of hemofilter, and stenosis [65]. Thrombosis is the most common reason for loss of access to the patient's circulation. Hypotension and hypovolemia during CRRT occur more frequently than with adults due to the smaller blood volume in children. Slower ultrafiltration rates reduce the risk of hypotension and circuit blood clotting. Other complications may include hypotension due to excessive fluid removal without appropriate fluid replenishment, hemorrhage due to over-anticoagulation, underlying cardiac dysfunction and electrolytes, and acid–base imbalances.

During therapy, meticulous monitoring of machine performance and of the patient's electrolytes and hemodynamics is required to prevent complications. Common problems include hypotension, arrhythmias, fluid balance and electrolyte disturbances, nutrient losses, hypothermia, and bleeding complications from anticoagulation. Continuous renal replacement therapy can result in clinically significant hypokalemia and hypophosphatemia, which may lead to severe complications if uncorrected.

The decision to terminate CRRT is made by the nephrologist or an experienced intensive care physician based on the patient's status recovery or decision of the patient and family.

The main indications for ceasing treatments to change a filter and the circuit relate to the status of the circuit and the vascular catheter access. These are measured by recording the different pressures within the circuit.

The following are the main indications for ceasing treatment:

1. The pre-filter pressure is consistently above 270 mmHg.
2. The transmembrane pressure is consistently above 250 mmHg.
3. The filter is over 72 h old.

If you troubleshoot these indications with no improvement, it is better to return the patient's blood from the circuit before total occlusion occurs so as not to inadvertently lose blood volume.

Hypotension

Hypotension during CRRT is usually secondary to intravascular volume depletion or underlying cardiac dysfunction.

Air Embolus

In current CRRT systems, the presence of air in the venous system will cause an alarm. When the alarm sounds, a clamp is engaged on the venous/return side to prevent the patient from receiving an air embolus. Blood leak alarms will be activated if the filter fibers split, causing blood to be lost in the ultrafiltrate compartment. Most systems also have malfunction or error codes that may signal during priming or therapy to indicate a problem with the system. These are specific to the system in use and providers should refer to their reference manuals to troubleshoot these alarms.

Cardiac Arrest

Cardiac arrest can result from air embolism, circulatory overload, arrhythmias, hypotension/hypertension, and/or hemolysis.

CRRT Outcome

Children with AKI requiring CRRT exhibit 40–50 % survival. Infants >3.0 kg has similar survival rates as older children [39, 58, 66–79]. Protracted periods of anuric or catabolic AKI often lead to the development of uremic syndrome. Most mortality occurs within 3 weeks of pediatric intensive care unit (PICU) admission. Children with increased degrees of fluid overload at CRRT initiation may develop pericarditis and pericardial effusion, anorexia, nausea, vomiting, ileus, and central nervous system disturbances, including lethargy, confusion, stupor, coma, agitation, focal neurological deficit, and seizures.

A retrospective study by Goldstein et al. examined outcome in 22 pediatric patients receiving CRRT and controlled for patient severity of illness using the pediatric risk of mortality (PRISM) score [2]. Neither means PRISM scores at the time of PICU admission nor time of CRRT initiation differed between survivors and non-survivors. Of the clinical variables studied (GFR, number of vasopressors, mean airway pressure, patient size, or % fluid overload), only the degree of % fluid overload at the time of CRRT initiation differed between survivors (16.4 ± 13.8 %) and non-survivors (34.0 ± 21.0 %, $p = 0.03$), even when controlled for severity of illness by PRISM score using a multiple regression model. This supports earlier data by Fargason et al. suggesting that the PRISM score may not be predictive [40]. A database by Bunchman et al. examined 226 children treated with RRT (CRRT, HD, and PD) looking at predictors of outcome. Diagnosis in these groups varied from AKI to inborn error of metabolism, to intoxications. Similar to adult data, outcome appears to be related not to age, not to modality but to severity of illness (i.e., vasopressor requirement) and underlying cause of need for RRT. This points out that it is not the modality but rather the underlying cause of the need for HF, as well as the overall hemodynamic status of the patient (including the presence or absence of vasopressor agents), that affects outcome. In children on CRRT and ECMO, outcome is primarily related to the need for extracorporeal membrane oxygenation (ECMO) and not to the use of CRRT. More recent single-center data, as well as multicenter data from the prospective pediatric CRRT registry group, support earlier findings that fluid overload at CRRT initiation is an independent risk factor for mortality in pediatric patients who receive CRRT.

Management of Electrolyte Imbalances During CRRT

Electrolyte imbalances are often due to high ultrafiltration rates, inadequate replenishment of electrolytes by intravenous infusion, or inadequate replenishment of bicarbonate loss during CRRT.

Azotemia

Increase replacement fluid flow rate.

Hyponatremia

Add 70 mL 3 % saline L to a 5-L bag.

Hypernatremia

Give electrolyte-free water by increasing peripheral infusion of 5 % dextrose or 0.45 % saline (1 L).

Metabolic Acidosis

Administer 100 mL of 50 % sodium bicarbonate iv infusion over 1 h, and you may repeat the dose PRN or alternatively you may change the replacement fluid to 5 % dextrose water and add 3 amps of sodium bicarbonate (50 %).

Metabolic Alkalosis

Change replacement fluid to 0.9 % saline and KCl sliding scale.

Hypercalcemia

Change bicarbonate dialysis (calcium-free) and increase replacement fluid rate or increase bicarbonate dialysate.

Hypocalcemia

Administer calcium chloride (10 %) 10 mL/100 mL 0.9 % saline or 5 % dextrose water over 1 h PRN.

Calcium Chloride (Ca^{++}) Infusion

Calcium chloride (Ca^{++}) infusion should be used with phosphorus solutions only. Add $CaCl_2$ 8 g in 1000 mL of 0.9 % NaCl and infuse in a central line other than hemofiltration access. The recommended infusion rate is 5 mg/kg/h to be given through the central line ONLY. Monitor the systemic ionized calcium level (from pre-filter) hourly until stable and then q6 h to adjust calcium infusion. Titrate $CaCl_2$ infusion to maintain patient Ca^{++} of 1.1–1.3 mmol/L (2.2–2.6 mg/dL) as shown below.

Patient Ca^{++} (mmol/L)	Ca^{++} infusion adjustment*
>1.3	Decrease rate by 10 mL/h
1.1–1.3 (optimum range)	No adjustment
0.9–1.0	Increase rate by 10 mL/h
<0.9	Increase rate by 20 mL/h
<0.8 or >1.3	Call nephrologists

*Notify MD if patient Ca^{++} <1 or if rate requires changes two times in 12 h
*Notify MD if calcium infusion rate >150 mL/h

Hypomagnesemia

Administer $MgSo_4$ (50 %) 2 mL in 100 mL 0.9 % saline or 5 % dextrose water over 1 h PRN. Follow the guidelines provided in Table 4.6 and monitor serum Mg^{++}level q2 h.

Magnesium Replacement

Follow the guidelines provided in Table 4.6 and monitor serum Mg^{++} level every 2 h.

Hypermagnesemia

Same as treatment for hypercalcemia.

Table 4.6 Magnesium (Mg^{++}) replacement during CRRT

Serum Mg^{++} level (mg/dL)	Mg^{++} dose (1.0 g/100 mL 5 % DW)
0.5–0.9	1.0 g/h × 3 doses
1.0–1.5	1.0 g × 2 doses
<0.5 or >2.5	Consult nephrologist

Hypophosphatemia

Follow the guidelines provided in Table 4.7 and monitor serum phosphate level q2 h.

Sodium Phosphate Replacement

Give an initial dose of sodium phosphate of 5 mL (3 mmol/mL) intravenously and follow the guidelines provided in Table 4.7.

Hypo- and Hyperkalemia

Follow the guidelines provided in Table 4.8, and monitor serum potassium level q2 h.

If hyperkalemia (serum potassium > 5.5 mEq/L), use potassium-free replacement solution and increase replacement and/or dialysate flow rate.

Table 4.7 Sodium phosphate (PO_4^-) replacement[a]

Serum PO_4^- level (mg/dL)	Sodium PO_4^- dose (mM/100 mL 5%DW)
1.5–1.9	30 mM (infuse at 10 mM/h)
2.0–2.5	20 mM (infuse at 10 mM/h)
<1.5 or >5.0	Consult nephrologist

[a]Repeat serum PO_4 level 2 h post-infusion

Table 4.8 Potassium replacement (mEq/L) during CRRT[a]

Serum K^+ level (mEq/L)	KCl dose (mEq)
3.2–3.5	20 mEq/k × 3 doses
3.6–3.9	20 mEq/h × 2 doses
4.0–4.2	20 mEq/h × 1 dose and 10 mEq/h × 1 dose
4.3–4.5	20 mEq/h × 1 dose
<3.2 or >5.4	Consult nephrologist

[a]Repeat potassium level 2 h post-infusion

References

1. Bunchman TE. Treatment of acute kidney injury in children: from conservative management to renal replacement therapy. Nat Clin Pract Nephrol. 2008;4:510–4.
2. Goldstein SL, Currier H, Graf JM, et al. Outcome in children receiving continuous hemofiltration. Pediatrics. 2001;107:1309–12.
3. Hayes LW, Oster RA, Tofil NM, Tolwani AJ. Outcomes of critically ill children requiring continuous renal replacement therapy. J Crit Care. 2009;24:394–400.
4. Ronco C, Parenzan L. Acute renal failure in infancy: treatment by continuous renal replacement therapy. Intensive Care Med. 1995;21:490–9.
5. Symons JM, Brophy PD, Gregory MJ, et al. Continuous renal replacement therapy in children up to 10 kg. Am J Kidney Dis. 2003;41(5):984–9.
6. Zhang YL, Hu WP, Zhou LH, Wang Y, Cheng A, Shao SN, Hon LL, Chen QY. Continuous renal replacement therapy in children with multiple organ dysfunction syndrome: a case series. Int Braz J Urol. 2014;40(6):846–52.
7. Zobel G, Kuttnig M, Ring E, Grubbauer HM. Clinical scoring systems in children with continuous extracorporeal renal support. Child Nephrol Urol. 1990;10:14–7.
8. Bunchman TE, Maxvold NJ, Brophy PD. Pediatric convective hemofiltration: Normocarb® replacement fluid and citrate anticoagulation. Am J Kidney Dis. 2003;42(6):1248–52.
9. Barenbrock M, Hausberg M, Marzkies F, et al. Effects of bicarbonate- and lactate-buffered replacement fluids on cardiovascular outcome in CVVH patients. Kidney Int. 2000;58:1751–7.
10. Bunchman TE, Maxvold NJ, Barnett J, et al. Pediatric hemofiltration: Normocarb® dialysate solution with citrate anticoagulation. Pediatr Nephrol. 2002;17:150–4.
11. Levraut J, Ciebiera JP, Jambou P, et al. Effect of continuous venovenous hemofiltration with dialysis on lactate clearance in critically ill patients. Crit Care Med. 1997;25:58–62.
12. Roy D, Hogg RJ, Wilby PA, et al. Continuous veno-venous hemodiafiltration using bicarbonate dialysate. Pediatr Nephrol. 1997;11(6):680–3.
13. Tobe SW, Murphy PM, Goldberg P, et al. A new sterile bicarbonate dialysis solution for use during cardiopulmonary bypass. ASAIO J. 1999;45(3):157–9.
14. Zimmerman D, Cotman P, Ting R, et al. Continuous veno-venous haemodialysis with a novel bicarbonate dialysis solution: prospective cross-over comparison with a lactate buggered solution. Nephrol Dial Transplant. 1999;14:2387–91.
15. Abramson S, Niles JL. Anticoagulation in continuous renal replacement therapy. Curr Opin Nephrol Hypertens. 1999;8:701–7.
16. Bellomo R, Teede H, Boyce N. Anticoagulant regimens in acute continuous hemodiafiltration: a comparative study. Intensive Care Med. 1993;19:329–32.
17. Favre H, Martin PY, Stoermann C. Anticoagulation in continuous extracorporeal renal replacement therapy. Semin Dial. 1996;9:112–8.
18. Fernandez SN, Santiago MJ, Lopez-Herce J, Garcia M, Del Castillo J, Alcaraz AJ, et al. Citrate anticoagulation for CRRT in children: comparison with heparin. Biomed Res Int. 2014;2014:786301. doi:10.1155/2014/786301. Epub 2014 Aug 3.
19. Mehta RL, Dobos GJ, Ward DM. Anticoagulation in continuous renal replacement procedures. Semin Dial. 1992;5:61–8.
20. Bihorac A, Ross EA. Continuous venovenous hemofiltration with citrate-based replacement fluid: efficacy, safety, and impact on nutrition. Am J Kidney Dis. 2005;46(5):908–18.
21. Chadha V, Garg U, Warady BA, Alon US. Citrate clearance in children receiving continuous venovenous renal replacement therapy. Pediatr Nephrol. 2002;17:819–24.
22. Egi M, Naka T, Bellomo R, et al. A comparison of two citrate anticoagulation regimens for continuous veno-venous hemofiltration. Int J Artif Organs. 2005;28(12):1211–8.
23. Maxvold NJ, Smoyer WE, Custer JR, Bunchman TE. Amino acid loss and nitrogen balance in critically ill children with acute renal failure: a comparison between CVVH and CVVHD therapies. Crit Care Med. 2000;28:1161–5.

24. Mehta RL, McDonald BR, Aguilar MM. Regional citrate anticoagulation for continuous arteriovenous hemodialysis in critically ill patients. Kidney Int. 1990;38:976–81.
25. Naka T, Egi M, Bellomo R, et al. Commercial low-citrate anticoagulation haemofiltration in high risk patients with frequent filter clotting. Anaesth Intensive Care. 2005;33(5):601–8.
26. Naka T, Egi M, Bellomo R, et al. Low-dose citrate continuous veno-venous hemofiltration (CVVH) and acid-base balance. Int J Artif Organs. 2005;28(3):222–8.
27. Tan HK, Uchino S, Bellomo R. Electrolyte mass balance during CVVH: lactate vs. bicarbonate-buffered replacement fluids. Ren Fail. 2004;26:149–53.
28. Brophy PD, Mottes TA, Kudelka TL, et al. AN-69 membrane reactions are pH-dependent and preventable. Am J Kidney Dis. 2001;38(1):173–8.
29. Lacour F, Maheut H. AN-69 membrane and conversion enzyme inhibitors: prevention of anaphylactic shock by alkaline rinsing? Nephrologie. 1992;13(3):135–6.
30. Brophy PD, Somers MJ, Baum MA, et al. Multicenter evaluation of anticoagulation in patients receiving continuous renal replacement therapy (CRRT). Nephrol Dial Transplant. 2005;20(7): 1416–21.
31. Chong BH, Magnani HN. Orgaran in heparin-induced thrombocytopenia. Hemostasis. 1992; 22:85–91.
32. Flanigan MJ, Von Brecht JH, Freeman RM, et al. Reducing the hemorrhagic complications of dialysis: a controlled comparison of low dose heparin and citrate anticoagulation. Am J Kid Dis. 1987;9:147–51.
33. Geary DF, Gajaria M, Fryer-Keeze S, Willemsen J. Low dose and heparin free hemodialysis in children. Pediatr Nephrol. 1991;5:220.
34. Kustogiannis DJ, Mayer I, Chin WD, et al. Regional citrate anticoagulation in continuous venovenous hemofiltration. Am J Kidney Dis. 2000;35:802–11.
35. Swartz RD, Port FK. Preventing hemorrhage in high-risk hemodialysis. Regional versus low-dose heparin. Kidney Int. 1979;16:513–8.
36. Elhanan N, Skippen P, Nuthall G, et al. Citrate anticoagulation in pediatric continuous venovenous hemofiltration. Pediatr Nephrol. 2004;19(2):208–12.
37. Liet JM, Allain-Launay E, Gaillard-LeRoux B, Barriere F, Chenouard A, Dejode JM, et al. Regional citrate anticoagulation for pediatric CRRT using integrated citrate software and physiologic sodium concentration solutions. Pediatr Nephrol. 2014;29(9):1625–31.
38. Macdonald D, Martin R. Use of sodium citrate anticoagulation in a pediatric continuous venovenous hemodialysis patient. ANNA J. 1995;22(3):21–4.
39. Tobe SW, Aujla P, Walele AA, et al. A novel regional citrate anticoagulation protocol for CRRT using only commercially available solutions. J Crit Care. 2003;18(2):121–9.
40. Fargason CA, Langman CB. Limitations of the pediatric risk of mortality score in assessing children with acute renal failure. Pediatr Nephrol. 1994;7:703–7.
41. Gainza FJ, Quintanilla N, Pijoan JI, Delgado S, Urbizu JM, Lampreeabe I. Role of prostacyclin (epoprostenol) as anticoagulant in continuous renal replacement therapies: efficacy, security and cost analysis. J Nephrol. 2006;19:648–55.
42. Hmiel SP, Martin RA, Landt M, et al. Amino acid clearance during acute metabolic decompensation in maple syrup urine disease treated with continuous venovenous hemodialysis with filtration. Pediatr Crit Care Med. 2004;5(3):278–81.
43. Kim HJ, Park SL, Park KI, Lee JS, Eun HS, Kim JH, et al. Acute treatment of hyperammonemia by continuous renal replacement therapy in a newborn patient with ornithine transcarbamylase deficiency. Korean J Pediatr. 2011;54(10):425–8.
44. McBryde KD, Kudelka TL, Kershaw DB, et al. Clearance of amino acids by hemodialysis in argininosuccinate synthetase deficiency. J Pediatr. 2004;144(4):536–40.
45. Meyer TW, Walther JL, Pagtalunan ME, et al. The clearance of protein bound solutes by hemofiltration and hemodiafiltration. Kidney Int. 2005;68(2):867–77.
46. Zappiteli M, Seymons JM, Somers MJG, et al. Protein and caloric intake prescription of children receiving continuous renal support therapy: a report from the prospective pediatric continuous renal support therapy registry group. Pediatr Crit Care Med. 2008;36:3239–45.

47. Zappitelli M, Juarez M, Castillo L, Cross-Bu J, Gildstein SL. Continuous renal replacement therapy amino acid, trace element, and folate clearance in critically ill children. Intensive Care Med. 2009;35:698–706.
48. Hackbarth RM, Eding D, Gianoli-Smith C, et al. Zero balance ultrafiltration (Z-BUF) in blood-primed CRRT circuits achieves electrolyte and acid-base homeostasis prior to patient connection. Pediatr Nephrol. 2005;20(9):1328–33.
49. Bunchman TE. Nutrition as medical therapy in pediatric critical illness. Clin J Am Soc Nephrol. 2013;8:513–4.
50. Davies SP, Reaveley DA, Brown EA, Kox WJ. Amino acid clearance and daily losses in patients with acute renal failure treated by continuous arteriovenous hemodialysis. Crit Care Med. 1991;19(12):1510–5.
51. Bambauer R, Inniger R, Pirrung KJ, et al. Complications and side effects associated with large-bore catheters in the subclavian and internal jugular veins. Artif Organs. 1994;18:318–21.
52. Bunchman TE, Gardner JJ, Kershaw DB, Maxvold NJ. Vascular access for hemodialysis or CVVH(D) in infants and children. Nephrol Dial Transplant. 1994;23:314–7.
53. Bunchman TE, Wilson SE, editors. Vascular access: principles and practice. 4th ed. Mosby: St. Louis; 2003. Pediatr Nephrol. 18(9):968.
54. Bunchman TE. Fluid overload in multiple organ dysfunction syndrome: a prediction of survival. Crit Care Med. 2004;32(8):1805–6.
55. Gillespie RS, Seidel K, Symons JM. Effect of fluid overload and dose of replacement fluid on survival in hemofiltration. Pediatr Nephrol. 2004;19(12):1394–9.
56. Jenkins R, Harrison H, Chen B, et al. Accuracy of intravenous infusion pumps in continuous renal replacement therapies. ASAIO J. 1992;38:808–10.
57. McBryde KD, Bunchman TE, Kudelka TL, et al. Hyperosmolar solutions in continuous renal replacement therapy for hyperosmolar acute renal failure: a preliminary report. Pediatr Crit Care Med. 2005;6(2):228–39.
58. Boschee ED, Cave DA, Garros D, Lequier L, Granoski DA, Guerra GG, et al. Indications and outcomes in children receiving renal replacement therapy in pediatric intensive care. J Crit Care. 2014;29:37–42.
59. Bouman CS, Oudemans-Van Straaten HM, Tissen JG, Zandstra DF, Kesecioglu J. Effect of early high-volume continuous venovenous hemofiltration on survival and recovery of renal function in intensive care patients with acute renal failure: a prospective, randomized trial. Crit Care Med. 2002;30(10):2205–11.
60. Chen CY, Tsai TC, Lee WJ, et al. Outcome prediction for critically ill children with acute renal failure requiring continuous hemofiltration. Renal Failure. 2004;26(4):35–9.
61. DiCarlo JV, Alexander SR, Agarwal R, Schiffman JD. Continuous veno-venous hemofiltration may improve survival from acute respiratory distress syndrome after bone marrow transplantation or chemotherapy. J Pediatr Hematol Oncol. 2003;25(10):801–5.
62. Elahi MM, Lim MY, Joseph RN, et al. Early hemofiltration improves survival in post-cardiotomy patients with acute renal failure. Eur J Cardiothorac Surg. 2004;26(5):1027–31.
63. Foland JA, Fortenberry JD, Warshaw BL, et al. Fluid over load before continuous hemofiltration and survival in critically ill children: a retrospective analysis. Crit Care Med. 2004;32(8):1771–6.
64. Bellomo R, Honroe PM, Matson J, et al. Extracorporeal blood treatment (EBT) methods in SIRS/sepsis. Int J Artif Organs. 2005;28:450–8.
65. Ricci Z, Guzzo I, Picca S, Picardo S. Circuit lifespan during continuous renal replacement therapy: children and adults are not equal. Crit Care. 2008;12(5):178.
66. Askenazi DJ, Goldstein SL, Chang IF, et al. Management of a severe carbamazepine overdose using albumin enhanced continuous venovenous hemodialysis. Pediatrics. 2004;113:406–9. POISOING.
67. Askenazi DJ, Feig DI, Graham NM, et al. 3–5 year longitudinal follow-up of pediatric patients after acute renal failure. Kidney Int. 2006;69:184–9.

68. Braun MC, Welch TR. Continuous venovenous hemodiafiltration in the treatment of acute hyperammonemia. Am J Nephrol. 1998;18(6):531–3.
69. Deodato F, Boenzi S, Rizzo C, et al. Inborn errors of metabolism: an update on epidemiology and on neonatal-onset hyperammonemia. Acta Paediatr Suppl. 2004;93(445):18–21.
70. Flores FX, Brophy PD, Symons JM, Fortenberry JD, Chua AN, Alexander S, et al. Continuous renal replacement therapy after stem cell transplantation. A report from the prospective pediatric CRRT registry group. Pediatr Nephrol. 2008;23(4):625–30.
71. Goldstein SL, Somers MJ, Baum M, et al. Pediatric patients with multi-organ system failure receiving continuous renal replacement therapy. Kidney Int. 2005;67(2):653–8.
72. Lane PH, Mauer SM, Blazar BR, et al. Outcome of dialysis for acute renal failure in pediatric bone marrow transplant patients. Bone Marrow Transplant. 1994;13:613–7.
73. McBryde KD, Kershaw DB, Bunchman TE, et al. Renal replacement therapy in the treatment of confirmed or suspected inborn errors of metabolism. J Pediatr. 2006;148(6):770–8.
74. Mehta RL, McDonald B, Gabbai FB, et al. A randomized clinical trial of continuous versus intermittent dialysis for acute renal failure. Kidney Int. 2001;60(3):1154–63. OUTCOME.
75. Metnitz PG, Krenn CG, Steltzer H, et al. Effect of acute renal failure requiring renal replacement therapy on outcome in critically ill patients. Crit Care Med. 2002;30:2051–8.
76. Meyer RJ, Brophy PD, Bunchman TE, et al. Survival and renal function in pediatric patients following extracorporeal life support with hemofiltration. Pediatr Crit Care Med. 2001;2:238–42.
77. Palmieri TL. Complication of continuous renal replacement therapy in children: are all created equal? Crit Care. 2010;14(1):105.
78. Picca S, Dionisi-Vici C, Abeni D, et al. Extracorporeal dialysis in neonatal hyperammonemia: modalities and prognostic indicators. Pediatr Nephrol. 2001;16(11):862–7. OUTCOME.
79. Piccinni P, Dan M, Barbacini S, et al. Early isovolaemic haemofiltration in oliguric patients with septic shock. Intensive Care Med. 2006;32(1):80–6. OUTCOME.

Chapter 5
Pharmacokinetics of CRRT

Drug Removal During CRRT: Basic Principles

Appropriate drug dosing in the acute kidney injury (AKI) patient treated with continuous renal replacement therapies (CRRT) is an important consideration to optimize therapeutic outcomes and to minimize drug toxicity [1–3]. Underdiagnosed and untreated AKI may lead to chronic kidney disease and end-stage renal disease [4]. When adjusting drug doses for the AKI patient, drug doses should be adjusted based on the renal and CRRT clearance of the drug, the degree of renal impairment, and the potential nephrotoxicity of the prescribed drug. The sum of renal creatinine clearance and CVVH ultrafiltration provides a starting point for subsequent antibiotic dosing. Medication dosing for children with AKI needs to be individualized based on pharmacokinetics and pharmacodynamics principles of the prescribed drugs whenever possible [5–11]. Both the volume of distribution and half-life of several drugs are markedly increased in the presence of AKI, and thus larger loading doses may need to be administered to achieve the target serum concentration. It is also necessary to know the degree of protein binding and the half-life of the concerned drug. Because of the presence of a positive fluid balance in the early stages of AKI, the dosing regimen for many drugs, especially antimicrobial agents, should be initiated at normal dosage regimens. When available, therapeutic drug monitoring should be used, especially for drugs with low therapeutic index. Guidelines whether or not dose adjustment is required for children with AKI is provided in Table 5.1.

The study of drug effects in human includes "pharmacokinetics" or the processes by which the body takes in, distributes, and disposes of a drug and "pharmacodynamics" which refers to the processes by which the drug has its desired effect [5–11]. For critically ill patients with renal failure, drug disposition is likely to be altered from what is observed in healthy volunteers, and consequently, the ability of a particular dosing regimen to achieve therapeutic goals in an individual patient may vary considerably from what the clinician expects.

F. Assadi, F.G. Sharbaf, *Pediatric Continuous Renal Replacement Therapy*,
DOI 10.1007/978-3-319-26202-4_5

Table 5.1 Pediatric drug dosage adjustments during continuous veno-venous hemofiltration (CVVH)[a]

Drug category	Protein binding (%)	SC	V_d L/kg	$t_{1/2}$ h	Normal dose (GFR 100)	Dose in CVVH <1–2 L/h GFR < 15–30
Analgesic						
Acetaminophen	20–50	0.93	0.2–0.4	2–3	5 mg/kg iv q8h	No change
Acetylsalicylic	>99	50	0.25	0.8	10 mg/kg q4–6h	No change
Codeine	7	NA	3–6	3	0.5–1 mg/kg q6h	75 % dose reduction
Ibuprofen	90–99	NA	0.14	1.8	5–10 mg/kg q6h	No change
Ketorolac	>99	NA	0.1–0.3	5	0.25–1 mg/kg q6h	No change
Fentanyl	80–85	0.29	2.4	2.6	1–5 mcg/kg q6h	75 % dose reduction
Meperidine	60–85	NA	2.4	11	0.5–2 mg/kg infusion	75 % dose reduction
Methadone	60–90	NA	4.5	8–49	0.5 mg/kg q6h	0.5 mg/kg q24h
Morphine	20–35	0.65	3.3	2.5	0.05–0.2 mg/kg iv q2–4h	75 % dose reduction
Antibiotics						
Aciclovir	9–33	0.85	0.7	2–3	10 mg/kg iv q8h	Normal dose iv q24h
Amikacin[b]	<20	0.95	0.2–0.7	1.6-2.5	20 mg/kg (max 1.5 g) iv q24h	10 mg/kg iv q24h
Amoxicillin	15–20	0.85	1.3	5–20	5–15 mg/kg iv q8h	No change
Amphotericin liposomal	90	NA	0.1–0.4	6–10	3–5 mg/kg iv q24h	No change
Ampicillin	17–20	0.8	0.32	1–1.8	50 mg/kg iv q8h	No change
Azithromycin	10–50	NA	NA	6–8	5 mg/kg q12	No change
Aztreonam	50–60	NA	0.25	2	80–120 mg/kg q8h	No change
Benzylpenicillin	60	NA	0.3–0.4	0.5–1.2	25–50 mg/kg iv in q8h	No change
Cefaclor	20–50	NA	0.24–0.35	1	10–20 mg/kg iv q12h	No change
Cefazolin	70–86	NA	0.13–0.22	2	50–100 mg/kg iv q8h	505 dose reduction
Cefotaxime	40	NA	0.3	1.5	50 mg/kg iv q8–12h	No change
Ceftazidime	<10	NA	0.2–0.4	1	25 mg/kg iv q8h	No change
Ceftriaxone	85–95	0.66	0.35	8	80 mg/kg (max 2 g) iv q24h	No change
Cefuroxime	33	0.66	0.19	1.5	25–50 mg/kg iv q8h	25–50 mg/kg iv q12–24 h
Cidofovir	<10	NA	0.3	15–25	5 mg/kg iv q 1–2 weeks	2 mg/kg iv q1-2 weeks

(continued)

Table 5.1 (continued)

Drug category	Protein binding (%)	SC	V_d L/kg	$t_{1/2}$ h	Normal dose (GFR 100)	Dose in CVVH <1–2 L/h GFR<15–30
Ciprofloxacin	20–40	0.7	2–3	4–5	10 mg/kg (max 400 mg) iv q12h	25 % reduction q 12 h
Clindamycin	>90	0.4	0.6–1.2	2–3	5–10 mg/kg (max 1.2 g) iv q6h	No change
Co-amoxiclav (amoxicillin + clavulanic acid)	17–30	NA	0.2–0.4	0.9	30 mg/kg (max 1.2 g) iv q8h	50 % dose reduction
Co-trimoxazole (trimethoprim + sulfamethoxazole)	50–66	NA	0.3–2.2	5.5–17	40–60 mg/kg ivq12h	50 % dose reduction
Erythromycin	70–95	0.3	0.6–1.2	2	12.5–25 mg/kg iv q6h	No change
Flucloxacillin	95	NA	0.13	2–3	25–100 mg/kg iv q8h	No change
Fluconazole	12	NA	0.6–1.2	15–20	6–12 mg/kg iv q72h	No change
Ganciclovir	1–2	0.84	0.4–0.8	3–28	5 mg/kg iv q12h	50 % dose reduction
Gentamicin[b]	1–30	0.95	0.2–0.5	1–3	7 mg/kg iv q24h	4 mg/kg iv q24h
Imipenem	13–21	1	0.5	1–1.3	15 mg/kg (max 500 mg) iv q6h	25 % dose reduction
Isoniazid	10–15	NA	NA	2.8	10–15 mg/kg q12–24h	No change
Ketoconazole	85–99	NA	2–4	8	3–6 mg/kg q24h	No change
Levofloxacin	25–38	0.8	NA	NA	5–10 mg/kg q24h	No change
Meropenem	2	NA	0.4	1.5–2.3	10–20 mg/kg iv q8h	No change
Metronidazole	<20	0.8	1.1	6–12	7.5 mg/kg (max 500 mg) iv q8h	No change
Nafcillin	90	0.2	0.35	1	15–50 mg/kg iv q4–6h	No change
Flaxacillin	20–30	NA	NA	NA	15 mg/kg iv q12h	No change
Piperacillin	20–30	NA	0.2	0.7	200 mg/kg q4h	200 mg/kg q8h
Rifampicin	80	0.2	0.66	1–3.8	10 mg/kg (max 500 mg) iv q12h	No change
Streptomycin	34	NA	NA	5–8	20–40 mg/kg iv q24h	7.5 mg/kg q24h
Ticarcillin	45–65	NA	0.22	1.1	80 mg/kg (max 3.2 g) q8h	No change
Tobramycin	44–50	1.6	1.6	11	60 mg/kg iv q12h	50 % dose reduction

(continued)

Table 5.1 (continued)

Drug category	Protein binding (%)	SC	V_d L/kg	$t_{1/2}$ h	Normal dose (GFR 100)	Dose in CVVH <1–2 L/h GFR < 15–30
Vancomycin[b]	55	NA	0.4–0.7	5.6	15 mg/kg iv q8h	10 mg/kg iv q12h
Anticoagulants						
Heparin[c]	95	<0.1	1	2	10–25 U/kg/h	No change
Warfarin	>90	0.02	0.05	50	0.5–8 mg q24h	No change
Anticonvulsants						
Carbamazepine	75–90	74	0.25	1.3	5–10 mg/kg q12h	75 % dose reduction
Phenobarbital	30–50	0.6	0.8	80	3–7 mg/kg q24h	10 mg/kg q 6-8 h
Phenytoin	80–90	0.1	0.6	20	3–7 mg/kg q8h	No change
Valproic acid	80–93	0.1	0.2–1	9–16	10–30 mg/kg q12h	No change
Antihistamines						
Cimetidine	19	0.8	1	2	4–8 mg/kg q12h	50 % dose reduction
Diphenhydramine	78	NA	3–6	5–11	1 mg/kg q4–6h	No change
Famotidine	15–20	NA	1–1.5	2–4	0.5 mg/kg q12h	No change
Terbutaline	25	NA	1.6	5.7	0.1–0.4 mg/kg/min iv infusion	No change
Antihypertensive agents						
Amlodipine	93	NA	21	40	0.05–0.17 mg/kg q24h	No change
Captopril	30	NA	1.5	1.5	0.1–0.5 mg/kg q6–8h	75 % dose reduction
Clonidine	20–40	0.7	2.1	8	2.5–5 mcg/kg q12h	No change
Enalapril	<50	0.5	1.7	11	0.1 mg/kg q12h	75 % dose reduction
Hydralazine	85–90					0.15 mg/Kg q8h
Isradipine	95	0.13	1.5	1	0.05–0.2 mg/kg q8h	No change
Labetalol	50				0.4–3 mg/h iv infusion	No change
Lisinopril	25	NA	NA	5–6	0.1 mg/kg q12–24h	0.50 % dose reduction
Nifedipine	95 %	0.08	1.2	2.8	0.25–0.5 mg/kg q6–8h	No change
Prazosin	95	0.03	0.6	2.9	0.2–1 mg/kg q12h	No change
Propranolol	60–90	0.07	4.3	3.5	0.1–1 mg/kg q6h	No change
Cardiovascular agents						
Amiodarone	96	0.03	61	N/A	5–10 mg/kg q24h	No change

(continued)

Table 5.1 (continued)

Drug category	Protein binding (%)	SC	V_d L/kg	$t_{1/2}$ h	Normal dose (GFR 100)	Dose in CVVH <1–2 L/h GFR<15–30
Atenolol	<5	1	0.43	6	1–2 mg/kg q24h	No change
Atropine	14–22	0.5	2.9	2–4	0.5–1 mg q5–30min	No change
Digoxin	20–55	0.8	6.5	40	250 mcg q24h	62.5 mcg q24h
Dobutamine	NA	NA	0.2	2	2–20 mcg/kg/min iv infusion	No change
Dopamine	NA	NA	NA	5.5	2–20 mcg/kg/min iv infusion	No change
Epinephrine	N/A	NA	<0.1	<0.1	0.01–1 mcg/kg/min iv infusion	No change
Milrinone	70	NA	0.38	2.3	0.25–0.75 mcg/kg/min iv infusion	0.33 mcg/kg/min iv infusion
Procainamide	15–20	NA	1.7–2.5	3–4	20–80 mcg/kg/min iv infusion	No change
Verapamil	90	0.13	4.3	5	1–2 mg/kg q8h	No change
Miscellaneous						
Aminophylline	40	0.47	NA	40	2 mg/kg q8h	No change
Cytoxan[d]	13	0.83	0.78	7.5	Follow protocol	50–75 % dose reduction
Cyclosporine[b, d]	96	0.1	3	1	Follow protocol	No change
Dexamethasone	68	0.32	1	3	1–4 mg q6h	No change
Hydrocortisone	70–90	NA	0.4–0.7	1.7	2–10 mg/kg q6h	No change
Insulin	98	0.95	<0.1	0.3	0.5–10 U/h	No change
Mycophenolate	97	NA	91	8–16	600 mg/m^2 q12h	No change
Sirolimus	92	NA	20	60	1 mg/m^2 q24h	No change

[a]References [3, 5–22]. Subsequent doses should be based on the estimated ultrafiltration capacity of the CVVH. *CVVH* continuous veno-venous hemofiltration, *SC* sieving coefficient (fraction), V_d volume distribution, $t_{1/2}$ half-time, *GFR* glomerular filtration rate, *iv* intravenous, *NA* not available
[b]Levels need to be checked daily
[c]Dose need to be adjusted according to APPT measured q12–24 h
[d]According to protocol

Absorption

Enteric drug absorption in the critically ill patient may be quite unpredictable for several reasons: proton-pump inhibitors administered for ulcer prophylaxis may raise gastric pH enough to dissolve pH-dependent coatings on tablets; fluid overload and gut edema as well as loss of enteric microarchitecture may impair absorption across the enteric mucosa; cholestasis in the setting of shock or sepsis may alter enterohepatic recirculation; disruption of epithelial tight junctions, loss of enteric mucosa, or partial denudation of the enteric lumen may lead to increased absorption; and first-pass effects may be altered by portosystemic shunts. For these reasons, oral administration of pharmacologic agents frequently is not even discussed in reviews of drug dosing in critical illness. Parenteral administration generally means intravenous infusion, although intraperitoneal and intrathecal administration may be preferred in certain settings.

Distribution

After an agent is administered—either orally or parenterally—it will be transported to a greater or lesser extent from its original location, namely, blood, CSF, and ascites, throughout the rest of the body. For this discussion, we will assume intravenous administration. As a result of this active and passive transport, the measured concentration of drug in the plasma will be less than just the administered dose divided by the estimated plasma volume. The dose administered divided by the final concentration yields a number with units of volume, called the "volume of distribution." It can be helpful in dose calculation to frame drug distribution in this way, even though the volume of distribution does not correspond to any particular anatomic space in the body. Once the drug has distributed throughout the body, it will have some final concentration and then gradually decrease as the body eliminates the drug. It may be challenging to distinguish drug excretion or metabolism from delayed distribution.

Unfortunately, the nomenclature is not entirely consistent in describing volume of distribution, and so it is worth some discussion here. Almost all drugs will exist in equilibrium between free drug—the active form of the drug—and drug that is specifically and nonspecifically bound to plasma and tissue proteins. Some drugs also partition into lipids. Often, descriptions of drug concentration and volume of distribution are not clear whether they are referring to both free and bound forms ("total drug") or the active, free form alone. An example familiar to most practicing nephrologists illustrates the point. Phenytoin, a commonly used antiepileptic, is highly protein bound to albumin (>90 %), and the total drug has a relatively small volume of distribution—about 0.7 L/kg in adults. The free, pharmacologically active form of the drug is thus only about 10 % of the total drug and circulates at a therapeutic concentration of 1–2 μg/mL. The volume of distribution for the free, active form of the drug is quite different (7 vs. 0.7 L/kg) from the volume distribution for the total drug, and the exact concentration of free drug is exquisitely sensitive to plasma protein concentrations and also, relevant for CKD and AKI, uremic toxins [5–11]. For this discussion, volume of distribution will refer to the free drug, not protein- and tissue-bound forms. A few other examples of drug distribution familiar to the practitioner from everyday experience may be helpful in anchoring the discussion. At one end of the spectrum, monoclonal antibodies, such as infliximab, are large molecules that are almost entirely retained in plasma and have very low volumes of distribution [4, 14]. In contrast, antimetabolites used in cancer chemotherapy are small molecules that bind extensively and nearly instantly to tissues and have volumes of distribution in the hundreds of liters [20, 22, 23].

The time course for transport of a drug depends on its chemical characteristics, especially size and protein binding, as well as the nature of the tissues into which it distributes. This matters not only in optimizing dosing strategies for the site of infection, but half-lives are affected by distribution, as reservoirs of drug in tissues may refill the plasma compartment as the kidney or liver removes the drug. Blood flow distributions to splanchnic nerve, skeletal muscle, and fat are altered in AKI and critical illness, so the apparent volume of distribution may change over the dosing cycle as well over the course of the illness. This effect may be modeled as early, nearly instant drug distribution into a "central" compartment and then slower distribution into one or more peripheral compartments. It is tempting but inaccurate to assign the identities of the modeled peripheral compartments to a particular organ or fluid. Drugs do not distribute into the entire body, and there are certainly anatomic compartments in the body to which some antibiotics have poor access, such as abscesses, bone, and CSF. Many antibiotics administered intravenously penetrate the blood–brain barrier slowly or not at all. This is a major challenge in therapeutic drug monitoring as antibiotic concentrations for therapeutic drug monitoring are usually measured in blood samples and almost certainly overestimate concentrations at the site of infection [7, 10].

Volumes of distribution in AKI may be severely deranged from published population estimates derived from healthy subjects [11, 13, 16–18]. First, hospitalized in-patients may have been obese and far above the ideal body weight at the time of admission, leading to overestimation of total body water if weight-based nomograms are used. Subsequent fluid overload and extracellular fluid volume expansion in turn increase volumes of distribution for hydrophilic drugs, such as aminoglycosides. Acutely ill subjects frequently have decreased plasma protein concentrations, and, additionally, uremic solutes such as hippurate and indoxyl sulfate alter drug binding to albumin in chronic renal failure and might do so in acute renal failure, although this has not been tested. The free fraction of many drugs—phenytoin, digoxin, and others—is increased in renal failure, even though the volume of distribution for total drug may increase due to movement of unbound drug into interstitial or total body water. Failure to adjust drug doses to account for these changes can result in unexpected toxicity as total drug remains the same, but the free concentration is higher than expected.

Creatinine clearance, commonly used as an easily calculated surrogate for glomerular filtration rate, includes creatinine removed from blood by glomerular filtration and tubular secretion, although in individual patients the relative contributions of each are generally not known. The same is true for drugs that may be filtered and either reabsorbed or secreted by the tubule. In renal failure, filtration and secretion are reduced, and it is usually assumed that reduced renal drug clearance occurs in proportion to reductions in glomerular filtration rate.

In consideration of drug clearance, metabolism of the drug is usually significant and sometimes dominates disappearance of drug from plasma. Metabolism may take the form of chemical modification of the drug by catalysis or hydrolysis or addition of groups that enhance excretion of the drug by modifying its solubility. The drug may also be secreted in bile and then eliminated unchanged in stool. Non-renal drug disposition is not independent of renal failure, however. Uremia and azotemia change hepatobiliary drug metabolism, possibly via product inhibition by accumulated metabolites. Hepatic cytochrome P450 expression is reduced in chronic uremia, and in vitro studies of rodent hepatocytes suggest that a dialyzable factor contributes to the suppression.

Extracorporeal clearance by the dialysis circuit occurs in parallel with endogenous clearance. Only the dialysis circuit removes the unbound or free drug, as the plasma proteins (albumin) to which the drug is bound are too large to pass through the pores of the dialysis membrane. CRRT has dialysate/effluent flow-limited small solute clearance (blood flow "Qb" ≫ dialysate flow "Qd"), and CRRT urea clearance is generally close to the effluent flow rate, typically 2–3 L/h or 33–50 mL/min. Peritoneal dialysis (PD) is only rarely used in acute renal failure, and drug kinetics in acute PD are not well studied. In CRRT, SLED, and conventional hemodialysis, middle molecule clearance is appreciably less than urea clearance and may be negligible.

Typical antibiotic dosing adjustments in CRRT involve estimating ongoing extracorporeal clearance (e.g., 15 mL/min) and dosing the antibiotic according to the guidelines for the equivalent creatinine clearance. Typical adjustments to dose in intermittent dialysis involve estimating drug removal in the course of a single session, frequently from the published literature rather than individualized data, and then supplementing the regular antibiotic dosing schedule with additional doses after each dialysis session. Anecdotal evidence suggests that individual institutions vary widely in their adherence to supplemental dosing.

The pharmacokinetics of drug removal in critically ill patients receiving CRRT is very complex, with multiple variables affecting clearance [1, 3, 6]. These variables make generalized dosing recommendations difficult [2, 4, 11, 14, 22, 23]. Drug–protein complexes have a larger molecular weight; therefore, antibiotics with low protein-binding capacity in serum are removed by CRRT more readily [9, 19, 21]. Similarly, antibiotics that penetrate and bind to tissues have a larger volume of distribution, reducing the quantity removed during CRRT [11, 13, 16–18, 24]. Sepsis itself increases the volume of distribution, extends drug half-life, and alters the protein-binding capacity of many antimicrobials. CRRT mechanical factors may also affect drug clearance. Increasing the blood or dialysate flow rate can change the transmembrane pressure and increase drug clearance. The dialysate concentration may also affect drug removal in hemofiltration. Lastly, the membrane pore size is directly proportional to the degree of drug removal by CRRT, often expressed as a sieving coefficient. Generally, biosynthetic membranes have larger pores, which allow removal of drugs with a larger molecular weight, unlike conventional filters. These patient, drug, and mechanical variables significantly diminish the utility of routine pharmacokinetic calculations for determining antimicrobial dosing during CRRT [7, 10].

Certain drugs are not dialyzable including dixogin, tricyclic, antidepressants, phenytoin, benzodiazepines, beta-blockers (atenolol is removed), and metformin.

Antimicrobial antibiotics fall into several broad classes of agent, which exert their selective effect on microbes by targeting enzymes that are not shared with their mammalian host. Each class of agent is thought to have a particular preferred concentration–time profile that optimizes microbial killing while minimizing side effects. Drugs are usually classed as time-dependent, meaning that time—or percentage of the dosing interval—above some threshold concentration influences kill rates to a greater extent than does the magnitude of the peak concentration observed; conversely, concentration-dependent agents show more dependence on the magnitude of the peak concentration than how long the concentration exceeded some multiple of the microbial minimum inhibitory concentration. Several agents exhibit a potent post-antibiotic or post-antifungal effect caused by the irreversible binding of the drug to bacterial or fungal cellular machinery. The pharmacokinetic processes (distribution and clearance) described above cause the concentration–time profile at the site of infection to differ from the concentration–time curve in plasma, so that plasma concentrations may or may not be close to concentrations at the site of infection. Optimization of the plasma concentration profile to achieve a desired tissue concentration–time profile is an active area of research.

Drug Dosing During CRRT

CRRT parameters substantially influence drug clearance. The mode of therapy (diffusion, convection, or both) can be influential, as both therapy modes can remove small solutes, but convective therapies are superior at removing larger solutes [10]. Drug clearance is affected by where replacement fluids are given, because this influences the drug concentration within the filter. Mathematical calculations can account for this, but published studies do not always specify this information. Filter composition can also influence drug removal. Some degree of drug adsorption occurs with many CRRT membranes (particularly sulfonated polyacrylonitrile and polymethylmethacrylate), although it is difficult to quantify adsorption in both in vitro and in vivo studies. Dialysis dose is one of the most influential factors, with increased dialysate/ultrafiltration/effluent flow rates resulting in greater drug removal [7]. Properties affecting drug removal during CRRT are different from those seen with intermittent hemodialysis. Therefore, dosing recommendations applicable for IHD would not be appropriate with these forms of therapy. In general, clearance properties of CRRT are dependent on the therapy utilized and on the pharmacokinetics/pharmacodynamics properties of each medication.

Drug removal during CRRT may occur by convection, diffusion, and adsorption. Convection and diffusion have the greatest influence on drug removal, while adsorption probably is less important, though it has not been studied widely. Drug removal is inversely proportional to the percentage of drug that is protein bound. If a drug is ≥80 % bound, little will be removed. This principle holds true for convection and diffusion. Ultrafiltration and dialysis flow rates (UFR/DFR) also affect drug clearance. Because CRRT uses highly permeable membranes, the molecular weight (MW) of most drugs has little impact on overall clearance. During convection, clearance of an unbound drug can be dramatic since CVVH can remove easily compounds with MW <15,000 Da. The impact of MW on drug removal during CVVHD is greater than the impact seen during CVVH. Solute clearance during CVVHD is dependent on diffusion, and, given that diffusion is inversely proportional to MW, the greatest impact is seen with drugs having a MW of <500 Da. Because many drugs used in the critical care setting have a MW of <500 Da, CVVHD can impact their removal significantly.

In order to devise a rational drug dosing regimen during CRRT, it is necessary to know the volume of distribution (V_d) and the clearance (CL) of the drug concerned [2, 5, 12, 15]. In the case of patients with AKI being treated with CRRT, clearance will depend on a combination of CRRT clearance, residual renal function, and non-renal clearance. Both the volume of distribution and the non-renal clearance may be changed by AKI and critical illness [8, 9, 13]. The problem is further exacerbated by considerable variability in the mode and dose of CRRT.

Drug dosing can be calculated from the knowledge of the pharmacokinetic parameters of a drug including the drug distribution, elimination within the body, and the desired drug plasma concentration.

Factors Influencing the Clearance of Drugs During CRRT

Drug removal during CRRT is determined by a complex interaction of many factors including the characteristics of the drug and the technical aspects of the CRRT (connective and diffusive) mechanism, the molecular size, protein binding, volume of distribution, water solubility, sieving coefficient, and plasma clearance [5, 8, 12, 15, 19]. When 25 % or more of an administered drug is removed by CRRT, it is considered clinically significant.

CRRT is dependent upon the use of a semipermeable membrane. The movement of drugs or other solutes is largely determined by the size of these molecules in relation to the pore size of the membrane. As a general rule, smaller-molecular-weight substances will pass through the membrane more easily than larger-molecular-weight substances [5, 8, 12, 15, 19].

Sieving Coefficient (SC)

Sieving coefficient is a useful tool to predict the likelihood of a drug across the CRRT membrane. Sieving coefficient is defined as the ability of a substance to pass through a membrane from the blood compartment of the hemofilter to the fluid compartment. Sieving coefficient is calculated as the ratio of drug concentration in the ultrafiltrate to the pre-filter plasma water concentration of the drug. The major determinant of the SC is the proportion of the plasma protein binding, because the drug that is bound to plasma protein is not available for filtration.

The SC values can vary from zero for drugs that cannot be filtered to one for drugs which are freely filtered. If the sieving coefficient is close to 1.0, the drug has relatively free passage across the filter; but at a coefficient of 0, the substance is unable to pass. Because the molecular weight cutoff for CRRT membrane is >20,000 Da, most low- and middle-molecular-weight substances have sieving coefficient of 1 [5, 10, 12, 15]. The sieving coefficient of sodium is 0.94, potassium 1.0, creatinine 1.0, and albumin 0.

Protein Binding

Another important factor determining drug clearance is the concentration gradient of unbound (free) drug across the CRRT membrane. Drugs with a high degree of protein binding will have a low plasma concentration of unbound (free) drug available for dialysis. The drug–protein complex is often too large to pass the hemodialysis membrane. Protein-bound drugs are largely inactive.

Plasma protein binding is a key determinant of V_d. Drugs that are highly protein bound will stay in the vascular space and have a low V_d. Protein-bound drugs are largely inactive.

Protein-binding drugs may increase or decrease in uremic patients with AKI.

Reduced plasma protein binding may result in freer drug available at the site of drug action/toxicity. Organic acids that accumulate in AKI will compete with acidic drugs (salicylate, warfarin, sulfonamides, phenytoin) for protein binding, and a larger fraction of acidic drugs will be available in the vascular space. Total and unbound (free) plasma phenytoin concentrations should be measured when monitoring drug dosages during CRRT. Basic drugs will bind more readily to non-albumin proteins, and there may be increased protein binding.

Low blood albumin concentration will result in decreased binding and more active free drug. Thus, protein binding is decreased in patients with nephrotic syndrome and is increased during albumin administration [5, 10, 12, 15].

Volume of Distribution

Volume of distribution (V_d) is the volume of plasma that would be necessary to account for the total amount of intravenously administered drug in the patient's body, if that drug were present throughout the body at the same concentration as found in the plasma. This value is usually further divided by the patient's body weight and the results expressed in terms of liters per kilogram (L/kg) [5, 10, 12, 15]. The volume of distribution (V_d) can be calculated by the following equation:

$$V_d\left(\text{L / kg body weight}\right) = \text{Amount of the drug administered}\left(\text{mg / kg}\right) \\ / \text{drug plasma concentration}\left(\text{mg / L}\right)$$

$$\text{Loading dose}\left(\text{LD}\right) = \text{dose}\left(\text{mg / kg}\right) / \text{concentration}\left(\text{mg / L}\right)$$

Therefore, the dose required to give a desired plasma concentration can be determined if the volume distribution for that drug is known. A drug with a large volume of distribution is distributed widely throughout the tissues and is present in relatively small amounts in the blood. Factors that contribute to a large volume of distribution include a high degree of lipid solubility and low plasma binding. Drugs, which have a large V_d, will eventually be cleared at a slower rate.

Drugs that are highly protein bound will stay in the vascular space and have a low volume of distribution. Lipid-soluble drugs, such as diazepam, or highly tissue-bound drugs, such as digoxin, have very high V_d. Lipid-insoluble drugs, such as neuromuscular blockers, remain in the blood and have a low V_d. Extracellular volume overload may increase the apparent V_d of highly water-soluble drugs, thus usual doses may result in low plasma levels in volume-overloaded patients. Extracellular volume contraction as well as muscle-wasted patients on the other hand has decreased apparent V_d and thus higher plasma levels.

Half-Life

Half-life ($t_{1/2}$) is the time in hours that it takes for the serum concentration of a drug to be reduced by 50 %. It is a function of plasma clearance and V_d.

Half-life ($t_{1/2}$) = 0.693 × ke h^{-1}, where ($t_{1/2}$) is the time in hours that it takes for the serum concentration of a drug to be reduced by 50 % and Ke h^{-1} = V_d (L) × CL (mL/min). Drug $t_{1/2}$ increases in oliguric AKI and shock syndromes. The longer drug $t_{1/2}$ in AKI may be a result of increased V_d and decreased clearance [5, 10, 12, 15].

Antibiotic Dose Adjustments

Because of the presence of a positive fluid balance in the early stages of AKI, the dosing regimen for many drugs, especially antimicrobial agents, should be initiated at a larger loading dose based on the expected volume of distribution to achieve the target serum concentration, and no adjustments need to be made for residual renal function.

Half-life ($t_{1/2}$) = 0.693 × ke h^{-1}, where ($t_{1/2}$) is the time in hours that it takes for the serum concentration of a drug to be reduced by 50 % and ke h^{-1} = V_d(L) × CL (mL)/min. Drug $t_{1/2}$ increases in oliguric AKI and shock syndromes [5, 10, 12, 15, 25].

Water Solubility

The dialysate used for CRRT (CVVHD and CVVHDF) is an aqueous solution. In general, drugs with high water solubility will be removed to a greater extent than those with high lipid solubility. High lipid-soluble drugs tend to be distributed throughout tissues, and therefore only a small fraction of the drug is present in plasma and accessible for dialysis [5, 10, 12, 15].

Plasma Clearance

Clearance of a drug is the volume of plasma from which the drug is completely removed per unit of time. The amount eliminated is proportional to the concentration of the drug in the blood. In dialysis patients, drug metabolism is unpredictable. Non-renal elimination, such as hepatic metabolism, may compensatorily increase, remain unchanged, or decrease.

In consideration of drug clearance, metabolism of the drug is usually significant and sometimes dominates elimination of drug from plasma. The drug may also be secreted in bile and eliminated in stool. Drug clearance [Cl] (mL/min) = volume (mL)/time (min), where Cl = describes clearance of drug (volume) from the body per unit time in min. Drug clearance decreases in patients with oliguric AKI.

The sum of renal and non-renal drug clearance is often termed the "plasma clearance" of a drug. In CRRT patients, renal clearance is largely replaced by CRRT clearance. If non-renal drug clearance (hepatic clearance) is large compared to renal clearance, the contribution of CRRT to total drug removal is low [5, 10, 12, 15].

CRRT Membrane

The characteristics of dialysis membrane determine to a large extent the clearance of drugs. Pore size, surface area, and geometry are the primary determinants of the performance of a given membrane [3, 4, 7, 13–15, 25]. In general, the molecular weight cutoff for the CRRT currently available membrane is >20,000 Da. A CRRT membrane with a larger surface area and greater permeability provides greater solute transfer and ultrafiltration. The surface area of the membrane should approximate the child's surface area under CRRT. The dialysis membrane constructed with polysulfone and polymethylmethacrylate membranes causes less pro-inflammatory cytokine activation than those constructed with cellulose or cuprophane.

Blood and Dialysate Flow Rates

The CRRT prescription includes the desired blood and dialysate flow rates. As drugs move from blood to dialysate, the flow rates of these two substances may have a significant effect on a drug clearance. In general, increased blood flow rates during CRRT will deliver greater amounts of drug to the CRRT membrane [22]. As the drug concentration increases in the dialysate, the flow rate of the dialysate solution also becomes important in overall drug removal. Higher dialysis can be achieved with faster flow rates that keep the dialysate drug concentration at a minimum [9].

CRRT Impact on Pharmacokinetic Parameters

AKI affects both distribution and elimination of many drugs [2, 9, 10]. CRRT also impacts on pharmacokinetic parameters in many ways. The wide variation in CRRT modalities may change drug removal and dosing in different settings.

CVVH uses a predominantly hydrostatic pressure gradient to pump solute across a filter membrane to achieve clearance. Replacement fluid can be added to the circuit either before blood reaches the membrane (pre-dilution) or after passage over the filter membrane (post-dilution). In contrast, CVVHD uses diffusion across a membrane to effect clearance of solute. This is achieved by generating a continuous concentration gradient using countercurrent flow of plasma and dialysate fluid, between which equilibration occurs. CVVHDF uses a combination of the two above techniques, convection and diffusion, to clear solute.

In general, the extent of drug removal is expected to be directly proportional to the hemofilter's surface area and to be dependent on the mode of replacement fluid administration (pre-dilution or post-dilution) and on the ultrafiltration and/or dialysate flow rates applied. Conversely, drug removal by means of CVVH or CVVHDF is unaffected by the drug size, considering that almost all antimicrobial agents have molecular weights significantly lower (<2000 Da) than the hemofilter cutoff (30,000–50,000 Da). Drugs that normally have high renal clearance and that exhibit high clearance during CVVH or CVVHDF may need a significant dosage increase in comparison with renal failure or even IHD. Conversely, drugs that are normally cleared and that exhibit very low clearance during CVVH or CVVHDF may need no dosage modification in comparison with normal renal function. Bearing these principles in mind will almost certainly aid the management of antimicrobial therapy in critically ill patients undergoing CRRT, thus containing the risk of inappropriate exposure. However, some peculiar pathophysiological conditions occurring in critical illness may significantly contribute to further alteration of the pharmacokinetics of antimicrobial agents during CRRT (i.e., hypoalbuminemia, expansion of extracellular fluids, or presence of residual renal function). Accordingly, therapeutic drug monitoring should be considered a very helpful tool for optimizing drug exposure during CRRT.

Replacement fluids may affect drug removal by influencing the drug concentration within the filter [23] Drug removal is also affected by filter result in membrane composition. Combined therapies (connective plus diffusive) provide greater drug removal by increasing dialysate/ultrafiltration/effluent flow rates. Furthermore, the drug dosing is further complicated by extracorporeal drug clearance on the altered pharmacokinetics caused by severity of illness and failure of several other organs.

Usual circuit priming volume ~100–150 mL can increase V_d. Tubing and membrane filter bind drug and increase V_d. The use of higher blood flow rate (>3–5 mL/kg/min) can also lead to increased CL. The use of higher ultrafiltration rate ~ filter replacement fluid rate (>35–40 mL/kg/h or 2.5 L/m^2/h) and higher dialysate rate (>35–40 mL/kg/h or 2.5 L/m^2/h) also lead to increased Cl. CRRT modalities on the other hand decrease drug ($t_{1/2}$) and will require dose adjustment to prevent toxicity and to ensure efficacy.

The correct drug dosing should consider not only the extracorporeal drug removal type of filter membrane but also residual renal and non-renal clearance and drug molecular weight, protein binding information, and volume of distribution to avoid medications error [3].

The ideal drug to be removed by CRRT that requires a dose adjustment has a low protein binding, a low volume of distribution, and a low non-renal clearance.

A simple and easy method for estimating drug clearance as a function of total creatinine clearance when the information on the pharmacokinetic of a particular drug is not available is to add replacement fluid rate (CVVH) or dialysate flow rate (CVVHD), usually 2 L/1.73 m^2/h or 33 mL/1.73 m^2/min, to the patient's native estimated creatinine clearance mL/1.73 m^2 (Schwartz formula). This value is the patient's new creatinine clearance and drug dose accordingly. This approach works in most cases and is good enough for initial dose estimates.

Drug Dosage Adjustments in CRRT

A quick look at the pharmacokinetic (absorption, distribution, elimination) sections of a drug monograph can help the practitioner quickly decide if renal dose adjustment is necessary. Once the practitioner has identified that renal clearance is a dominant or mechanism of elimination, he or she needs to estimate the aggregate renal and extracorporeal drug elimination in his or her individual patient. Typical dose adjustments categorize renal function roughly into <10 mL/min, 10–20 mL/min, 30–60 mL/min, or >60 mL/min; many variations on this theme exist, but the concept is uniform. Renal clearance can be assumed to be nearly zero in anuric patients, and in patients with some urine output, a rapid assessment of function with a 4-h creatinine clearance can broadly assign a patient's renal function to one of the categories in the dosing guide.

There is little if any data to support reduction of the initial antibiotic dose solely on the basis of renal failure; the most obvious influences on the volume of distribution of the free drug tend to cancel each other: hypoalbuminemia tends to increase the free fraction of drug, while extracellular fluid volume expansion dilutes that free fraction more than in a normovolemic patient. Aminoglycosides and vancomycin will continue to require weight-based dosing and therapeutic drug monitoring wherever possible. The more complicated aspect of dosing lies in scheduling subsequent doses. Concentration-dependent agents, such as fluoroquinolones, aminoglycosides, daptomycin, and amphotericin, generally are adjusted by altering the length of the dosing interval, whereas for time-dependent agents such as beta-lactams and triazoles, the dosing interval is kept constant or nearly so, and the dose is reduced. Individual hospitals' prescribing practices often combine both approaches.

By aggregating measured renal and calculated extracorporeal clearance into a single number, the practitioner has a surrogate for creatinine clearance that allows application of the more commonly available dose adjustments for chronic kidney disease to patients with AKI with or without residual renal function and any renal replacement strategy, bearing in mind that most drugs undergo multiple clearance mechanisms, and this approach only accounts for the renal component of clearance.

Drug dosing for septic patients with acute renal failure receiving continuous renal replacement therapy (CRRT) is complicated, and failure to correctly dose may result in either drug toxicity or treatment failure and development of antibiotic resistance.

In order to devise a rational drug dosing regimen, it is necessary to know the volume of distribution (V_d) and the clearance (CL) of the drug concerned. In the case of patients with ARF being treated with CRRT, clearance will depend on a combination of CRRT clearance, residual renal function, and non-renal clearance. Both the volume of distribution and the non-renal clearance may be changed by ARF and critical illness. The problem is further exacerbated by considerable variability in the mode and dose of CRRT. Thus, to be useful to clinicians, studies of antibiotic pharmacokinetics in critically ill patients with ARF should report several parameters in addition to the standard pharmacokinetic dataset. Without these parameters, interpretation of studies and their use in deriving a dosing regimen are limited.

We conducted a comprehensive review of Medline-referenced literature to formulate dosing recommendations for the drugs frequently used to treat clinically ill adults and pediatric patients undergoing CRRT [3, 5–22].

We used these data, as well as clinical experience, to make recommendations for antibiotic dosing in critically ill children treated with CVVH. For drugs with no specific published data on dosing in children receiving CVVH, we used known chemical properties and other clinical data (e.g., protein-binding capacity, sieving coefficient, volume of distribution, half-life) to make initial dosing recommendations (Table 5.1). Subsequent dosing should be based on the estimated ultrafiltration capacity of the CVVH.

The pharmacokinetics and pharmacodynamics properties of each listed drug were considered. However, these recommendations are meant to serve only as a guide until more data are available. Table 5.1 provides guidelines for drug dosage adjustments in children receiving CVVH therapy.

Loading Dose (LD)

Loading doses are useful for drugs that are eliminated from the body relatively slowly. These drugs need only a low maintenance dose in order to keep the amount of the drug in the body at the target level. Without loading, it would take longer for the amount of the drug to reach target level. Three variables are used to calculate the loading dose including desired peak concentration of drug (CP), V_d, and drug bioavailability (F). The required loading dose may then be calculated as

$$\text{Loading dose}(\text{mg / kg}) = V_d \times \text{CP}(\text{mg / L}) \times \text{body weight}(\text{kg}) / F.$$

For an intravenously administered drug, the bioavailability F will equal 1, since the drug is directly introduced to the bloodstream. If the patient requires an oral dose, bioavailability will be less than 1 (depending upon absorption and metabolism), requiring a larger loading dose.

Loading doses typically are adjusted based on V_d and are not adjusted for renal failure. If extracellular volume depletion is present, V_d may be reduced and reductions in loading dose should occur.

Maintenance Dose

Maintenance doses ensure steady-state blood concentrations and lessen the likelihood of subtherapeutic regimens or overdoses. In the absence of a loading dose, maintenance doses will achieve 90 % of their steady-state level in 3–41⁄2 lives.

Maintenance dose can be calculated as follows:

$$\text{Maintenance dose}(\text{MD})\,\text{mg} = \text{CL}(\text{mL / min}) \times \text{serum concentration}(\text{mg / mL}) \times \text{dosing interval}(\text{min})$$

Antimicrobial Agents

Antibiotic selection and dosing are often challenging in critically ill patients because of disease complexity, resulting in physiological alterations and reduced antibiotic susceptibilities of nosocomial pathogens and may result in either underdosing, causing treatment failure and antibiotic resistance, or overdosing resulting in drug toxicity.

This is further compounded by the use of renal replacement therapy (RRT) to maintain homeostasis until renal function has sufficiently recovered, which can result in significant non-renal clearance of antibiotic.

Most antibiotics require a dose adjustment in patients receiving CRRT. Many drugs have a narrow therapeutic window. Pharmacokinetic parameters already discussed may alter the way antimicrobials are handled or excreted. For orally administered agents, decreased absorption or co-binding will occur if administered with antacids or phosphorus binders. Loading doses typically are the same; however, most maintenance doses will have a longer interval.

Depending on the drug, it may be more appropriate to shorten the dosing interval or to increase the dose. For example, in oliguric AKI patients, a very small single daily dose of aminoglycosides can be used to achieve peak concentrations and to avoid toxic side effects. After CRRT initiation, it is recommended to increase the single daily dose to achieve peak levels while lowering aminoglycosides levels to low trough concentration and avoiding the risk of side effects. In contrast, the bactericidal effect of β-lactam antibiotics (penicillins and cephalosporins) correlates with constant plasma levels above the minimal inhibitory concentrations of the bacteria, and side effects may occur if high peak concentrations are reached with the use of high single doses. In these drugs, it may be useful to shorten the dosing intervals instead of increasing the individual dose.

Although early and appropriate antibiotic therapy remains the most important intervention for successful treatment of septic shock, data guiding optimization of beta-lactam prescription in critically ill patients prescribed with CRRT are still limited.

Optimization of beta-lactam therapy in CRRT is complex and is dependent on several drug, CRRT, and patient-related factors. Consideration of drug properties and protein binding, CRRT settings, and disease-related pharmacokinetic alterations is essential for individualizing dose regimens with the purpose of attaining pharmacodynamics targets associated with success.

All β-lactams are of small size (molecular weight <800 Da) and have volume distributions >0.3 L/kg and protein bounding fraction <10 % except for oxacillin and ceftriaxone which are not clinically significant. They undergo significant extracorporeal clearance during CVVH [5, 8, 25]. Being small hydrophilic molecules, beta-lactams (meropenem, piperacillin, and ceftriaxone) are likely to be cleared by CRRT to a significant extent. As a result, additional variability may be introduced to the per se variable antibiotic concentrations in critically ill patients. For empirically optimized dosing, during the first day, an initial loading dose is required to achieve drug concentrations within the therapeutic range early in time, regardless of impaired organ function. An additional loading dose may be required when CRRT is initiated due to steady-state equilibrium breakage driven by clearance variation. From day 2, dosing must be adjusted to CRRT settings and residual renal function. Therapeutic drug monitoring of beta-lactams may be regarded as a useful tool to daily individualize dosing and to ensure optimal antibiotic exposure.

Meropenem and aminoglycosides also have pharmacokinetic properties such as low molecular weight, small volume of distribution, and negligible protein binding. They are easily filtered due to its low molecular weight, low volume of distribution, and low protein binding. In contrast, quinolones (ciprofloxacin and levofloxacin) with molecular weight about 370 Da, volume of distribution 1.2–1.8 L/kg, and protein binding of 25–50 % are less liable to clearance by CVVH [8, 20–22].

Glycopeptides (vancomycin) has a large molecular weight nearly 1550 Da with volume distribution of 0.38 L/kg and protein binding of 30 %. The normal functioning kidneys clear about 70 % of the drug. The clearance rates of vancomycin in patients on CAVVH are compatible with clearance in patients with GFR >50 mL/min [16].

Therapeutic vancomycin levels are difficult to maintain in critically ill patients who are receiving iv vancomycin therapy while on CRRT. Aggressive dosing schedules and frequent monitoring are required to ensure adequate vancomycin therapy in this setting.

Vancomycin serum levels are frequently insufficient in critically ill patients receiving CRRT. One possible strategy to optimize vancomycin therapy in this setting is to aim for 12 hourly dosing with serum level monitoring as early as 6–12 h after the first infusion followed by dynamic adjustment of dose and/or dosing intervals to maintain serum levels within therapeutic targets.

Aggressive dosing schedules and frequent monitoring are required to ensure adequate vancomycin therapy in this setting.

Monitoring drug levels is important. Peak level is usually obtained 30 min following iv dose and 60–120 min after oral ingestion. Trough level is obtained just prior to the next dose and may be used as a marker of drug toxicity.

Analgesics, Sedatives, and Psychotropic Drugs

Most nonnarcotic analgesics are metabolized by the liver, thus require little or no dosage adjustment in ESRD. AKI may increase the sensitivity to the pharmacologic effects of narcotics. Meperidine (Demerol) accumulates in patients with decreased GFR and may lower the seizure threshold. Morphine also accumulates and one should avoid repetitive dosing. Neuromuscular blocking agents are excreted by kidneys and may have a prolonged half-life in patients with ESRD.

Antidepressants such as tricyclic antidepressants should be used cautiously given the increased risk of adverse side effects. Lithium is water soluble with a small molecular weight and is easily removed with dialyzer.

Antihypertensive Agents

Most blood pressure-lowering medications can be safely prescribed in patients with AKI. Post-dialysis dosing or extra doses after dialysis may be necessary for certain antihypertensive agents:

1. Angiotensin-converting enzyme inhibitors (ACE-I): all are dialyzable except fosinopril
2. Angiotensin receptor blockers (ARB): none are dialyzed
3. B-blockers: atenolol and metoprolol are dialyzable, but labetalol and carvedilol are not
4. Calcium channel blocker: amlodipine is not dialyzable

Anticoagulants

Low-molecular-weight heparin will accumulate in patients with AKI and should not be used during CRRT. If used, follow anti-factor Xa levels and reduce the dosing interval.

Endocrine Drugs

Hypoglycemic agents that are excreted by the kidneys, such as sulfonylureas, should be not be used.

Rheumatologic

There is increased risk of adverse effects with allopurinol due to its metabolite. Colchicine has an increased risk of myopathy and polyneuropathy.

Anticonvulsants

The V_d of phenytoin is increased, while the degree of protein binding is decreased. Thus, total plasma drug levels may not reflect subtherapeutic drug levels, as the free level may be adequate. It is therefore, recommended to monitor both free and total phenytoin levels in AKI patients.

Vasopressors

Vasopressor agents (epinephrine, norepinephrine, dopamine, dobutamine) all have in common a small molecular weight and minimal protein binding and clear from plasma rapidly.

References

1. Aronoff GR, Bennett WM, Berns J, Brier ME, Kasabaker N, Mueller BA, Pasko DA, Smoyer WA. Drug prescribing in renal failure: dosing guidelines for adults and children. 5th ed. Philadelphia: American College of Physicians; 2007.
2. Assadi F. Medication dosing and renal insufficiency in a pediatric cardiac intensive unit. Pediatr Cardiol. 2008;29:1029–30.

3. Buckmaster JN, Davis AR. Guidelines for drug dosing during continuous renal replacement therapies. In: Ronco C, Bellomo R, editors. Critical care nephrology. New York: Springer; 1998. p. 1327–34.
4. Bunchman TE. Medication errors and patient complications with continuous renal replacement therapy. Pediatr Nephrol. 2006;21:842–5.
5. Bauer SR, Salem C, Connor Jr MJ, Groszek J, Taylor ME, Wei P, Tolwani AJ, Fissell WH. Pharmacokinetics and pharmacodynamics of piperacillin-tazobactam in 42 patients treated with concomitant CRRT. Clin J Am Soc Nephrol. 2012;7(3):452–7.
6. Bugge JF. Pharmacokinetics and drug dosing adjustments during continuous venovenous hemofiltration or hemodiafiltration in critically ill patients. Acta Anaesthesiol Scand. 2001;45(8):929–34.
7. Kuang D, Verbine A, Ronco C. Pharmacokinetics and antimicrobial dosing adjustment in critically ill patients during continuous renal replacement therapy. Clin Nephrol. 2007;67:267–84.
8. Reetze-Bonorden P, Böhler J, Keller E. Drug dosage in patients during continuous renal replacement therapy: pharmacokinetic and therapeutic considerations. Clin Pharmacokinet. 1993;24:362–79.
9. Roder BL, Frimodt-Moller N, Espersen F, Rasmussen SN. Dicloxacillin and flucloxacillin: pharmacokinetics, protein binding and serum bactericidal titers in healthy subjects after oral administration. Infection. 1995;23:107–12.
10. Subach RA, Marx MA. Drug dosing in acute renal failure: the role of renal replacement therapy in altering drug pharmacokinetics. Adv Ren Replace Ther. 1998;5:141–7.
11. Varghese JM, Jarrett P, Boots RJ, Kirkpatrick CM, Lipman J, Roberts J. Pharmacokinetics of piperacillin and tazobactam in plasma and subcutaneous interstitial fluid in critically ill patients receiving continuous venovenous haemodiafiltration. Int J Antimicrob Agents. 2014;43:343–8.
12. Bressolle F, Kinowski JM, de la Coussaye JE, Wynn N, Eledjam JJ, Galtier M. Clinical pharmacokinetics during continuous haemofiltration. Clin Pharmacokinet. 1994;26:457–71.
13. Carcelero E, Soy D. Antibiotic dose adjustment in the treatment of MRSA infections in patients with acute renal failure undergoing continuous renal replacement therapies. Enferm Infect Microbiol Clin. 2012;30(5):249–56.
14. Churchwell MD, Mueller BA. Drug dosing during continuous renal replacement therapy. Semin Dial. 2009;22(2):185–8.
15. Connor Jr MJ, Salem C, Bauer SR, Hofmann CL, Groszek J, Butler R, Rehm SJ, Fissell WH. Therapeutic drug monitoring of piperacillin-tazobactam using spent dialysate effluent in patients receiving continuous venovenous hemodialysis. Antimicrob Agents Chemother. 2011;55:557–60.
16. Covajes C, Scolletta S, Penaccini L, Ocampos-Martinez E, Abdelhadii A, Beumier M, Jacobs F, de Backer D, Vincent JL, Taccone FS. Continuous infusion of vancomycin in septic patients receiving continuous renal replacement therapy. Int J Antimicrob Agents. 2013;41:261–6.
17. Choi G, Gomersall CD, Tian Q, Joynt GM, Freebairn R, Lipman J. Principles of antibacterial dosing in continuous renal replacement therapy. Crit Care Med. 2009;37:2268–82.
18. Jamal JA, Economou CJ, Lipman J, Roberts JA. Improving antibiotic dosing in special situations in the ICU: burns, renal replacement therapy and extracorporeal membrane oxygenation. Curr Opin Crit Care. 2012;18:460–71.
19. Lau AH, Kronfol NO. Determinants of drug removal by continuous hemofiltration. Int J Artif Organs. 1994;17:373–8.
20. Veltri MA, Neu AM, Fivush BA, Parekh RS, Furth SL. Drug dosing during intermittent hemodialysis and continuous renal replacement therapy: special considerations in pediatric patients. Pediatr Drugs. 2004;6:45–65.
21. Vincent HH, Vos MC, Akcahuseyin E, Goessens WH, van Duyl WA, Schalekamp MA. Drug clearance by continuous haemodiafiltration: analysis of sieving coefficients and mass transfer coefficients of diffusion. Blood Purif. 1993;11:99–107.

22. Vos MC, Vincent HH, Yzerman EPF, Vogel M, Mouton JW. Drug clearance by continuous haemodiafiltration: results with the AN-69 capillary haemofilter and recommended dose adjustment for seven antibiotics. Drug Invest. 1994;7:315–22.
23. Keller F, Böhler J, Czock D, Zellner D, Mertz AKH. Individualized drug dosage in patients treated with continuous hemofiltration. Kidney Int. 1999;56 Suppl 72:S29–31.
24. Li AM, Gomersall CD, Choi G, Tian Q, Joynt GM, Lipman J. A systematic review of antibiotic dosing regimens for septic patients receiving continuous renal replacement therapy: do current studies supply sufficient data? J Antimicrob Chemother. 2009;64:929–37.
25. Choi G, Gomersall CD, Tian Q, Joynt GM, Freebairn R, Lipman J. Principles of antibacterial dosing in continuous renal replacement therapy. Blood Purif. 2010;30:195–212.

Chapter 6
Case Management

Below we have summarized our experience treating ten children with severe AKI complicated by sepsis, hyperkalemia, diuretic-resistant fluid overload, inborn error of metabolism, and/or organ dysfunction syndromes (MODS) treated with CRRT. All ten recovered completely, thus supporting the effectiveness of CRRT for the management of children who are critically ill due to AKI complicated by MODS.

Case Study

A 4.5-year-old boy was admitted to pediatric intensive care unit (PICU) with a 3-day history of non-projectile vomiting and fever. The patient was also experiencing loss of consciousness on admission and suffered a convulsion on the day after admission, with a concomitant sustained decrease in blood pressure and urine output. His urine output was <1 mL/kg/h.

On examination, he had generalized edema, and his weight was 21 kg, temperature 40.1 °C, blood pressure 68/41 mmHg, respirations 19 breath/min, and heart rate 110 beats/min. He had MODS including AKI, disseminated intravascular coagulation, acute myocardial injury, acute liver injury, and meningitis.

Laboratory data included: white cell count (WBC) of 21.2×10^6/dL, hemoglobin (Hb) 9.2 g/dL, platelets 152×10^3/dL, sodium 129 mEq/L, chloride 101 mEq/L, potassium 5.6 mEq/L, calcium 8.5 mg/dL, phosphorus 6.1 mg/dL, BUN 54 mg/dL, and creatinine 4.5 mg/dL. Arterial blood gas (ABG) analysis showed pH 7.15, HCO_3^- 9 mEq/L, and pCO_2 32 mmHg. Liver function studies included alanine transaminase (ALT) 12,982 U/L, aspartate transaminase (AST) 14,782 U/L, total bilirubin 1.13 mg/dL, direct bilirubin 0.11 mg/dL, albumin 2.6 g/dL, creatinine kinase (CPK) 25175 U/L, C-reactive protein (CRP) 11 mg/dL, activated partial thromboplastin time (APTT) 65/s, prothrombin time (PT) 29.1/s, and international normalized ratio (INR) 5.74. Blood, urine, and spinal fluid cultures grew gram-positive staphylococcus bacteria. He was started on epinephrine infusion 4 μg/min

F. Assadi, F.G. Sharbaf, *Pediatric Continuous Renal Replacement Therapy*,
DOI 10.1007/978-3-319-26202-4_6

and phenobarbital for the management of hypotension and control of seizures, respectively.

Questions

1. Would CRRT be indicated?
2. What mode of therapy would be best for this patient and why?
3. Would you remove fluids?
4. When would you initiate treatment with CRRT?

Comments

Because of the altered mental status, hyponatremia, metabolic acidosis, electrolyte imbalance, oliguric AKI, and increased serum creatinine and CPK levels due to septic shock and hepatic failure, the patient underwent treatment with CRRT [1–13].

He was treated with meropenem and gentamicin during CVVH treatment for the bacterial infection according to the guidelines recommended in Table 4.7.

The patient underwent CRRT treatment for 256 h. His liver and renal function gradually improved. BUN, serum creatinine, and electrolyte levels normalized. His blood pressure and urine output normalized (1.5–1.7 L/24 h). He was discharged home 4 days after CRTT cessation.

CRRT Prescriptions

1. Treatment modality: CVVH
2. Machine: Prismaflex
3. Hemofilter: M60, AN69
4. Catheter: 8.5 Fr
5. Priming: 0.9 % saline
6. Vascular access: right internal jugular vein
7. Anticoagulation: heparin (first dose 450 units, maintenance dose 100–300 units/h); clotting time was maintained between 20 and 30 min and APTT was 1.5–2.0 times normal
8. Blood flow rate (BFR): 80 mL/min
9. Replacement fluid rate: bicarbonate-based solution, 750 mL/h using the post-dilution method
10. Dialysate flow rate: none
11. Fluid removal rate: 50–100 mL/h

He remained in the hospital for additional 6 days before discharge. After discharge, the patient was followed up once monthly for 12 months. His development was normal and there was no relapse of symptoms/biochemical abnormalities.

Case Study

A 5-week-old female neonate was transferred to the PICU because of MODS (congestive heart failure, AKI, lungs, hypoxic encephalopathy) due to neonatal asphyxia and meconium aspiration syndrome.

Upon admission to PICU, her temperature was 36 °C, respiration 26 breath/min, heart rate 123/beats/min, and blood pressure 65/42 mmHg. She weighed 3.7 kg and was 46 cm tall. Her daily urine output averaged <1.0 mL/kg/h.

Laboratory data included: WBC of 18.6 × 106/dL, Hb 14.2 g/dL, platelets 180 × 10 /dL, sodium 133 mEq/L, chloride 109 mEq/L, potassium 5.4 mEq/L, calcium 6.6 mg/dL, phosphorus 5.9 mg/dL, BUN 47 mg/dL, creatinine 5.3 mg/dL, ALT 496 U/L, AST 676 U/L, total bilirubin 1.42 mg/dL, direct bilirubin 0.62 mg/dL, albumin 3.1 g/dL, CRP 6 mg/dL, APTT 34/s, PT 16.3/s, and INR 1.32. ABG revealed pH 7.21, HCO_3^- 10 mEq/L, and pCO_2 29 mmHg. The chest film showed bilateral pulmonary infiltration with pleural effusion. Blood, urine, and spinal fluid cultures showed no bacterial growth.

The patient was electively intubated for airway protection and treated with gentamicin and ampicillin. The antibiotic doses were adjusted according to the recommendation provided in Table 4.7.

Questions
1. Would CRRT be indicated?
2. What mode of therapy would be best for this patient and why?
3. Would you remove fluids?
4. When would you discontinue treatment with CRRT?

Comments

CRRT treatment was initiated because of the neonatal oliguric AKI and MODS [9, 12–18].

CRRT Prescriptions
1. Treatment modality: CVVH
2. Machine: Prismaflex
3. Hemofilter: AN69, M60
4. Catheter: 7 Fr
5. Priming: blood
6. Vascular access: right jugular vein

7. Anticoagulation: no heparin
8. Blood flow rate (BFR): 30 mL/min
9. Replacement fluid rate: bicarbonate solution, 500 mL/h using the post-dilution method
10. Dialysate flow rate: none
11. Fluid removal rate: 15–50 mL/h

The patient's electrolytes and urine output gradually normalized. Her urine output rose to 600–750 mL/day. BUN and serum creatinine fell to 21 mg/dL and 1.2 mg/dL, respectively. The serum electrolytes returned to normal levels and her liver function improved. After discharge, the patient was followed up once monthly for 9 months. Her development was normal and there was no relapse of symptoms or biochemical abnormalities.

The patient underwent bedside CRRT treatment for 65 h and was hospitalized for additional 14 days before discharge. After discharge, the patient was followed up once monthly for 12 months. Her development was normal, and there was no relapse of symptoms/biochemical abnormalities.

Case Study

A 14-year-old boy was rushed to the hospital emergency department after rescued from a collapsed building for nearly 12 h. Emergency amputation of the right arm was performed due to severe crush injury. She developed MODS (heart failure, liver failure, respiratory distress syndrome, AKI, and disseminated intravascular coagulation) complicated with sepsis 2 days after the surgery.

On examination she was unconscious and edematous. Her weight was 36 kg, temperature 39.5 °C, heart rate 167 beats/min, respiration 14/min, and blood pressure 90/57 mmHg. Diffused rales and crackles were heard in both lungs. Purulent secretion was noticed at the amputation site. Many contusion wounds were seen over the entire body. The infant was intubated for airway protection (FiO_2 70 %) and treated with antibiotics.

Laboratory tests showed: WBC $18{,}204 \times 10^6$/L, Hb 6.8 g/dL, Hct 19 %, and platelet count 45×10^6/L. Serum sodium was 131 mEq/L, potassium 6.8 mEq/L, chloride 98 mEq/L, bicarbonate 11 mEq/L, creatinine 5.3 mg/dL, BUN 67 mg/dL, total bilirubin 9.2 mg/dL, direct bilirubin 7.8 mg/dL, albumin 3.3 g/dL, ALT 230 IU/L, AST 651 IU/L, CK 8621 IU/L, myoglobin 5400 ng/mL, PT 20.1 s, APTT 120 s, and TT 45.2 s. Chest X-ray revealed bilateral pleural effusion. Blood, urine, spinal fluid, and wound cultures grew multiple pathogenic microorganisms including *Klebsiella pneumoniae*, *Staphylococcus aureus*, and *Staphylococcus epidermidis*, which were treated with meropenem plus vancomycin. The antibiotic doses were adjusted according to the recommendations provided in Table 4.8.

Questions

1. Would CRRT be indicated?
2. What mode of therapy would be best for this patient and why?
3. Would you remove fluids?
4. When would you discontinue treatment with CRRT?

Comments

CRRT treatment was initiated because of the AKI and MODS complicated with sepsis [9, 12–18].

CRRT Prescriptions

1. Treatment modality: CVVH
2. Machine: Prismaflex
3. Hemofilter: AN69, M100
4. Catheter: 8.5 F
5. Priming: 0.9 % saline
6. Vascular access: right internal jugular vein
7. Anticoagulation: regional citrate
8. Blood flow rate (BFR): 180–200 mL/min
9. Replacement fluid rate: 2000 mL/h
10. Dialysate flow rate: none
11. Fluid removal rate: 40 mL/kg/h with 65 % pre-dilution and 35 % post-dilution

The CRRT treatment was continued for 102 h. At this point, the patient's clinical status improved considerably. Her temperature was 38.1 °C, heart rate 98 beats/min, respiratory rate 17/min, and blood pressure 134/74 mmHg. Her urine output rose to 1.600–2.4 L/day. The patient's BUN and serum creatinine fell to 27 mg/dL and 1.5 mg/dL, respectively. The WBC decreased to 9.5×10^6/L and platelet count increased to 178×10^6/L. Serum electrolytes, liver function, and coagulation abnormalities returned to normal. She remained in the hospital for additional 16 days before discharge. After discharge, the patient was followed up once monthly for 12 months. His development was normal and there was no relapse of symptoms/biochemical abnormalities.

In all these cases, we believe that early intervention with CRRT may have inhibited the cytokine cascade/systematic inflammatory response and the associated inflammatory injury [7, 11]. The amelioration of uremia and fluid overload likely contributed to the efficacy of treatment [19–25].

CRRT treatment of 265 h for the first patient is relatively rare [26, 27]. This duration of treatment was necessary to stabilize the patient's internal environment, provide nutritional/metabolic support, and allow for the implementation of other supportive treatment. Cases 2 and 3 are unique because there have been few reports of survival in neonates with MODs and children with MODS and sepsis following the crush injury [15–17].

For these patients, an AN69 membrane filter M60 with good biocompatibility, high permeability, and strong adsorption capacity was used [28, 29]. The area of the filter was relatively large (0.6 m^2). The membrane, which can also be used under hypotension, causes a weak activation of complement and leukocytes and has a small impact on hemodynamics. The high permeability of this membrane may help to improve the anti-inflammatory cytokine to pro-inflammatory cytokine ratio, downregulate the body's inflammatory response, and ameliorate the systemic inflammatory response [11].

One of the keys to early intervention in the neonate was placement of a central venous catheter. The smallest M60 filter was used and the tubing was prefilled with whole blood. Further, at the beginning of CRRT, the BFR was low, thus preventing a subsequent drop in blood pressure. Attention was also paid to body heat preservation and heating the vascular access point [4, 30–33].

Case Study

A 5-year-old girl with new onset AKI due to septic shock has pulmonary edema and hyperkalemia. She is intubated with a FiO_2 of 65 % and a peep of 10. Her laboratory studies showed sodium 170 mEq/L, potassium 6.5 mEq/L, BUN 78 mg/dL, creatinine 3.9 mg/dL, and osmolality 488 mOsm/L. A trial of loop diuretic failed to induce diuresis.

1. Which form of renal replacement (RRT) is most appropriate?
2. What are the patient's risk factors?
3. What is the osmolality of RRT solutions?

Which form of RRT is least efficient?

Comments

This patient benefits from CRRT (connective or diffusive) because of combination of volume overload, hyperkalemia, and increased serum osmolality in a setting of AKI complicated with an osmolality of ~285 mOsm/L. Thus, 3 % hypertonic saline must be added to CRRT solutions prior to the therapy to avoid disequilibrium syndrome [34].

CRRT yields the least efficient clearance (0.1–8 L/h) compared with peritoneal dialysis 0.5–2 L/h or hemodialysis 30–50 L/h.

Case Study

A 9.5-kg male infant presents with lethargy. The child is afebrile; blood pressure is 75/40 mmHg, heart rate 130 beats/min, and respirations 50/min. On examination he appeared lethargic and "floppy" with poor neurologic tone.

Laboratory data showed hemoglobin of 15; creatinine of 0.9 mg/dL, potassium of 4.3 mEq/dL, calcium of 9.5 mg/dL, phosphorus of 6.0 mg/dL (nL), bicarbonate of 14 mEq/L, and ammonia of 1533 μmol/L (normal <40 μmol/L).

The child was electively intubated for airway protection. Foley catheter was placed for urine collection. Arginine chloride (250 mg/kg/2 h followed by 250–500 mg/kg/day), carnitine (1.0 g iv bolus followed by 250–500 mg/kg/day), sodium phenylacetate/sodium benzoate (250 mg/kg/2 h + 250 mg/kg/day), vitamin B12 (1 mg), and biotin (10 mg) all began once urine and plasma for amino and organic acids were obtained.

1. What is you CRRT prescription
2. Would you remove fluids?
3. Will the CRRT therapy clear sodium phenylacetate and sodium benzoate?

CRRT Prescriptions

1. Treatment modality: CVVHD
2. Machine: CARPEDIEM
3. Hemofilter: AN69 membrane filter M60 (0.5 m^2)
4. Catheter: 7 Fr, 10 cm double lumen
5. Priming: wool blood
6. Vascular access: left internal jugular vein
7. Anticoagulation: regional citrate
8. Blood flow rate (BFR): 200 mL/min (~20 mL/kg/min)
9. Replacement fluid rate: 2 L/h
10. Dialysate flow rate: 1 L/h
11. Fluid removal rate: 40 mL/kg//h

Blood ammonia levels collected at 1 h intervals. At 6 h of CVVHD the ammonia was ~200 µmol/L.

Comments

Hyperammonemia is extremely toxic to the brain (per se or through intracellular excess glutamine formation) causing astrocyte swelling, brain edema, coma, death, or severe disability; thus, emergency treatment has to be started even before having a precise diagnosis since prognosis mainly depends on coma duration [10, 35].

Immediate institution of medical therapy is essential, and an early decision of CRRT institution is needed. Ammonia is non-osmolar so no risk of dialysate disequilibrium exists. Liver transplantation should be considered if medical and CRRT management is not successful.

Infants with inborn error of metabolism appear to be polyuric so keeping them intubated and keeping them "wet" is important. Sodium phenylacetate, sodium benzoate, and arginine, like ammonia, are low-molecular-weight compounds and nonprotein binding, and they will be removed during CRRT treatment [36, 37].

Case Study

You are consulted to see a 4-year-old admitted to the pediatric intensive care unit with vasopressin-dependent gram-negative septic shock secondary to community-acquired pneumonia. His medical condition is complicated by respiratory failure, pericardial rub, and oliguric AKI. His serum potassium is 6.6 mEq/L, creatinine 3.8 mg/dL, and BUN 63 mg/dL.

1. Would you start CRRT and why?
2. What mode of therapy would be best for this patient?
3. What is the mortality rate?

Comments

Sepsis is the most common cause of AKI in the ICU setting. The patient is hemodynamically instable. CRRT is indicated because of hemodynamic instability, AKI, acute respiratory failure, fluid overload, and hyperkalemia [1, 8, 35, 38]. CVVH (convection) is the preferred modality for septic AKI [3, 11, 39–41]. Convective removal of inflammatory mediators with molecular size <30,000 Da is likely with CVVH. In patients with AKI requiring CRRT, mortality ranges from 50 to 70 %.

Case Study

A 16-year-old male status post-bone marrow transplant for aplastic anemia was admitted to ICU for management of AKI complicated by pulmonary failure requiring mechanical ventilation, sepsis, and liver failure secondary to graft-versus-host disease (GVHD). CVVHD was initiated for management of multiorgan dysfunction syndrome (MODS), fluid overload, and hyperkalemia (K^+ 6.7 mEq/L) with electrocardiogram changes. He was treated with gentamicin 180 mg iv q24 h and vancomycin 1 g iv q24 h. Blood levels of gentamicin and vancomycin 12 h post-infusion were 3.8 mg/L and 21 mg/L, respectively, while dialysis rate was 1000 mL/h. The dialysis rate increased to 1200 mL/h, and repeat blood levels 12 h post-gentamicin and vancomycin infusion were <0.4 and <4 mg/dL.

1. Will the drugs be removed during CVVHD?
2. How often do you do drug dosage adjustments during CVVHD?

Comments

CRRT drug clearance is usually considered clinically significant only if its contribution to total body clearance exceeds 25–30 % [28, 42–49]. Factors that influence drug removal by CRRT include its membrane characteristics (permeability, sieving coefficient), CRRT modality (convection with or without diffusion), blood, replacement fluid, dialysate, and ultrafiltration flow rates as well as duration of CRRT.

The sieving coefficient is the capacity of a drug to pass through the hemofilter membrane. Only drugs not bound to plasma proteins can pass the filter and be removed by CRRT.

Gentamicin and vancomycin (protein binding <70–80 %, volume distribution <1 L/kg) will be removed by CVVHD [50–59].

Drug dose adjustments are required if the GFR during CVVH is 20–20 or 20–50 mL/min during CVVHD. Loading doses do not need to be adjusted because loading dose depends solely on volume of distribution. Recommendations for maintenance doses are listed on Table 4.8. Frequent blood level determinations are highly recommended during the course of CRRT.

We firmly believe that to ensure optimal CRRT for AKI patient in the ICU, the skills and the experience of the physicians and nurses who perform dialysis are more important than the applied dialysis modalities.

Case Study

A 17-year-old female, 60 kg, was admitted to ICU for acute peritonitis. She was rushed to the operating room because of an acute abdomen. On postoperative day 2, she became septic. Her blood pressure was 81/58 mmHg while on dopamine drips. Her urine output is <100 mL/day. She is intubated and is on mechanical ventilator. Serum creatinine and BUN levels were 6.1 and 87 mg/dL, respectively. WBC was 13.2×10^9/dL, HCT 30 %, platelet counts 156×10^3/dL, CRP 190 mg/dL, PTT 49 s, ACT 210 s, liver function normal, arterial blood pH 7.14, $PaCO_2$ 22.5, sodium 132 mEq/L, potassium 5.9 mEq/L, chloride 98 mEq/L, and bicarbonate 14 mEq/L.

1. What is the most appropriate renal replacement therapy (RTT) (peritoneal dialysis, intermittent hemodialysis, or CRRT) and why?
2. Which CRRT modality should be used and why?

Comments

The absolute indications for RRT are BUN >100 mg/dL, hyperkalemia <6 mEq/L with ECG abnormality, metabolic acidosis (pH<7.15) and lactic acidosis related to metformin use, and diuretic-resistant fluid overload. Anuria/oliguria (RIFLE class R, I, F), blood pH>7.15, BUN >76 mg/dL, hyperkalemia >6 mEq/L without ECG abnormality, and edema responsive to diuretics are considered relative criteria for the RRT initiation.

CRRT is a preferred RRT modality in this critically ill patient because of her multiorgan dysfunction syndrome [1–13].

CRRT Prescription

1. Modality: CVVH
2. Machine: Prismaflex
3. Hemofilter: M150, AN69
4. Catheter: 14 Fr, double lumen, 25 cm
5. Priming: 0.9 % saline + heparin 2500–500 unit/L
6. Vascular access: right femoral vein
7. Anticoagulation: low-dose heparin (initial bolus 5–10 units/kg, infusion at 31–12 units/kg/h)
8. Blood flow rate: 250 mL/min
9. Replacement fluid: bicarbonate-based post-dilution method 1.9 L/h.

   Solution 1: 1 L of 0.45 % saline + 7.5 % $NaHCO_3$ 90 mL + 50 % glucose 8 mL.

   Solution 2: 1 L of 0.4 % saline + 3 % saline 150 mL + 50 % $MgSO_4$ 0.5 mL + KCl 8 mEq/L.

Final concentration (mEq/L) Na = 138; K = 4.0; HCO_3 = 35; Mg = 1.0; glucose = 190)

10. Ultrafiltration rate, 2 L/h; net fluid removal rate, 100 mL/h
11. Calcium replacement: 10 % calcium gluconate (60 mL) + 5 % dextrose water (40 mL) drip at 10 mL/h
12. Monitoring: serum electrolytes, calcium, and glucose every 8 h and BUN creatinine, PO_4, Mg, CBC, ACT post-filter (180–240 s), PTT (45–55 s), and liver function test every 24 h.

Case Study

A previously healthy 2½-year-old girl was presented to the PICU with a 3-day history of high fever and erythematous rash and vesicles over her hands, feet, and mouth due to enterovirus 71-related hand, foot, and mouth disease. On examination she appeared lethargic with reduced consciousness. Her weight was 16.9 kg, temperature 40 °C per rectum, blood pressure 70/30 mmHg, heart rate 190 beats/min, and respirations 33 breath/min. The oxygen saturation was 78 % in room air. She had cool, mottled skin and a prolonged capillary refill time was noted. Results of arterial blood gas showed pH 7.25, pCO_2 40 mmHg, PO_2 81 mmHg, bicarbonate 12 mEq/L, and oxygen saturation 78 % in room air.

A chest X-ray showed bilateral pulmonary edema with normal heart size. Electrocardiography showed sinus tachycardia. Echocardiogram showed severe dilated left ventricular dilation. The central venous pressure was 5.8 cmH_2O. She immediately required endotracheal intubation and positive pressure ventilation support. Normal saline 20 mL/kg was given over 30 min with vasopressin infusion including dobutamine 0.4 μg/kg/min, epinephrine 0.5 μg/kg/min, and milrinone 15 μg/kg/min.

Laboratory investigations revealed the following values: WBC $17{,}600 \times 10^6$/L, neutrophils >10,000 × 10/L, lymphocyte 3110 × 106/L, hemoglobin 11.7 g/dL, platelet count 165×10^3/L, APTT 34 s, BUN 34 mg/dL, creatinine 1.1 mg/dL, glucose 98 mg/dL, sodium 124 mEq/L, potassium 5.6 mEq/L, chloride 98 mEq/L, bicarbonate 17 Eq/L, calcium 8.1 mg/dL, total bilirubin 2.1 mg/dL, aspartate aminotransferase 45 IU/L, alanine aminotransferase 3.8 IU/L, lactate dehydrogenase 534 IU/L, ammonia 56 mg/dL, C-reactive protein 3.2 mg/L, total protein 6.4 g/dL, and albumin 3.3 g/dL.

1. What mode of therapy would be best for this patient and why?
2. Outline the dosing of CRRT

Comments

CVVH was initiated 4 h after PICU admission because of pulmonary edema, refractory hypotension, septic shock syndrome, and cardiopulmonary failure.

CRRT Prescriptions

1. Modality: CVVH
2. Machine: Prismaflex
3. Hemofilter: M60, AN69
4. Catheter: 8 Fr, double lumen
5. Priming: 0.9 % saline + heparin 2500–500 unit/L
6. Vascular access: right internal jugular vein
7. Anticoagulation: heparin (initial bolus 5–10 units/kg, infusion at 31–12 units/kg/h)
8. Blood flow rate: 5 mL/kg/min (850 mL/min)
9. Replacement fluid: bicarbonate-based pre-filter method 60 mL/kg/h (1.0 L/h)
10. Ultrafiltration rate, 1.3 L/h; net fluid removal rate, 30 mL/h
11. Calcium replacement: 10 % calcium gluconate (60 mL) + 5 % dextrose water (40 mL) drip at 10 mL/h
12. Monitoring: serum electrolytes, calcium, and glucose every 8 h; BUN creatinine, PO_4, Mg, CBC, ACT post-filter (180–240 s), PTT (45–55 s), liver function test every 24 h

CVVH was sustained for 140 h without any complications. The patient's hemodynamic status became more stable with a heart rate of 120 beats/min and blood pressure of 110/62 mmHg. Vasopressors were discontinued. A cardiac ultrasound showed an improved left ventricular hypertrophy. She was discharged after 2 weeks of hospitalization without any obvious squeal.

Case Study

A 9-month-old (10 kg) boy was admitted to PICU for AKI, fluid overload, and severe hyperkalemia (6.9 mEq/L) with ECG abnormality following cardiac surgery for closure of ventricular septal defect. Laboratory data revealed the following values: WBC $14{,}100 \times 10^6$/L, Hct 30 %, platelet count 205×10^3/L, ACT 225 s, BUN 51 mg/dL, creatinine 1.3 mg/dL, glucose 101 mg/dL, sodium 138 mEq/L, potassium 6.9 mEq/L, chloride 99 mEq/L, bicarbonate 9 mEq/L, calcium 8.8 mg/dL, total bilirubin 1.1 mg/dL, aspartate aminotransferase 35 IU/L, alanine aminotransferase 3.0 IU/L, C-reactive protein 14 mg/L, total protein 6.1 g/dL, and albumin 3.9 g/dL.

CRRT was initiated because of AKI complicated with hyperkalemia and severe acidosis.

Prescriptions

1. Machine: Prismaflex
2. Hemofilter: M60, AN69
3. Catheter: 7 Fr, double lumen
4. Priming: 0.9 % saline + heparin 2500–500 unit/L
5. Vascular access: right internal jugular vein
6. Anticoagulation: heparin (initial bolus 5–10 units/kg, infusion at 5–12 units/kg/h)
7. Blood flow rate: 5 mL/kg/min (50 mL/min)
8. Replacement fluid: bicarbonate-based post-filter method 40 mL/kg/h (600 mL/h)
9. Ultrafiltration rate: 400 mL/h
10. Calcium replacement: 10 % calcium gluconate (60 mL) + 5 % dextrose water (40 mL) drip at 10 mL/h

Two episodes of filter thrombosis and circuit clotting occurred within the first 24 h of the CVVH initiation.

1. Where is the problem?
2. How do you repair the problem?

Comments

The problem with circuit clotting is due to low blood flow rate and post-filter administration of replacement fluid.

The actual amount of delivered blood flow is less than the administered blood flow.

The actual blood flow reaching the filter is 70 mL/min [(1-Hct) × administered blood flow rate (100 mL/min)] with filtration fraction of 24 % (ultrafiltration (17 mL/min)/delivered BFR (70 mL/min) × 100).

Replacement fluid was given as pre-dilution (pre-filter) and blood flow was increased to 150 mL/min (delivered BFR 105 mL/min (0.7 × 150)) and fraction filtration fell to 16 % (17/105 × 100).

However another early filter thrombosis observed.

What is wrong?

Consider replacing the existing catheter with a larger size and shorter length.

We believe that several reasons underlie this high rate of treatment success in our case series. First, the decision to treat with CRRT was made early [7, 35]. Second, CRRT allows for correction of water and sodium retention and electrolyte imbalances in a timely manner, facilitating the effectiveness of other treatments [19–25, 60, 61]. Finally, we must admit that involvement and cooperation between a multidisciplinary team are of paramount importance so that appropriate rescue of respiratory failure, use of breathing machines, infection prevention and treatment, and cardiovascular support can be accomplished.

With regard to when to withdraw treatment, we believe that CCRT can be ceased once water and sodium retention subsides, urine output returns to normal, and renal function recovers [5, 7].

Due to the physiological and anatomical characteristics of children, including low body weight, small blood flow volume, and hemodynamic instability, we recommend that a successful implementation of CRRT in children should take into account the following:

- There is a strong epidemiologic association between development of acute kidney injury and subsequent development and progression of chronic kidney disease [62, 63]. The epidemiologic association is seen across a broad array of clinical settings, with a graded risk with increased severity or increased number of episodes of acute kidney injury [64–68]. The link between acute kidney injury and subsequent chronic kidney disease is supported by experimental data demonstrating vascular rarefaction and activation of fibrotic pathways following acute kidney injury. Common risk factors for the development of both acute kidney injury and chronic kidney disease make it difficult to definitively establish a causal relationship on the basis of epidemiologic data [64–68].
- It is recommended to define AKI according to the RIFLE classification system into ARF risk, ARF injury, and ARF failure [69, 70].
- The diagnostic value of urinary biomarkers for early detection of AKI in newborns and children is well documented and is now available in most hospital laboratories [71–75].
- It is also recommended to base the decision when to start CRRT not only on the severity of ARF but also on the severity of other organ failure [5, 7, 9, 12, 13, 76, 77]. Initiation of CRRT is to be considered in oliguric patients despite adequate fluid resuscitation and/or a persisting steep rise in serum creatinine, in addition to persisting shock [5, 7, 76].
- Potential benefits of CRRT in patients with multiple organ dysfunctions include management of fluid balance, decreasing fluid overload, removal of inflammatory mediators, enhanced nutritional support, and control of electrolyte and acid–base abnormalities [11, 19–25].
- For cases involving AKI, particular attention should be paid to water and sodium retention and blood nitrogen levels, all of which have a significant impact on the treatment and survival of infants and young children, as well as the speed of progress. The characteristics of systemic disease are also an important factor.
- CRRP is an extracorporeal blood purification therapy intended to substitute for impaired renal function over an extended period of time and applied for 24 h a day [3, 15, 40]. CRRT requires a central double-lumen veno-venous hemodialysis catheter [30, 31, 78], an extracorporeal circuit and a hemofilter [79, 80], and a blood pump and an effluent pump. With specific CRRT therapies dialysate and replacement pumps are also required [81–87].

- SCUF requires a blood and an effluent pump but no dialysis or replacement solution is needed. Fluid removal up to 2 L can be achieved. The primary goal is safe management of large fluid removal via ultrafiltration [40].
- Ultrafiltration transport mechanism forces the movement of fluid through a semipermeable membrane driven by a pressure gradient. The effluent pump forces plasma water and solutes, to a small degree, across the membrane in the filter. This transport mechanism is used in SCUF, CVVH, CVVHD, and CVVHDF [88–90].
- CVVH requires blood, effluent, and replacement pumps [3, 91, 92]. Dialysate is not required. Plasma water and solutes are removed by convection and ultrafiltration.
- Convection transport mechanism removes middle and large molecular solutes as well as large volumes of fluid simultaneously. This transport mechanism is used in CVVH and CVVHDF.
- Bicarbonate-based or lactate-based replacement fluids are used (pre- or post-filter) based on the patient's clinical need. Higher replacement fluid rates increase convective clearances.
- CVVHD requires the use of blood, effluent, and dialysis pump. Replacement solution is not required. Plasma water and solutes are removed by combination of diffusion and ultrafiltration. Dialysate is used to create a concentration gradient across a semipermeable membrane. This transport mechanism is used in CVVHD and CVVHDF. Through diffusion, dialysate corrects underlying metabolic imbalances. Dialysate is dependent on buffering agent, electrolytes, and glucose concentrations. Dialysate composition should reflect normal plasma values to achieve homeostasis.
- Bicarbonate-based solution is physiologic and replaces lost bicarbonate immediately. A bicarbonate concentration of 30–35 mEq/L corrects metabolic acidosis in 24–48 h. It is a superior buffer in normalizing acidosis without the risk of alkalosis. Bicarbonate-based solution is also a preferred buffer for patients with liver failure. It improves hemodynamic instability with fewer cardiovascular events [81–83, 85–87].
- Lactate-based solution is metabolized into bicarbonate in the liver on a 1:1 in subjects with normal liver function and can sufficiently correct acidemia. However, lactate-based solution has a pH value of 5.4, and it is a powerful peripheral vasodilator leading to further acidemia for patients with hypoxia, liver impairment, and preexisting lactic acidemia [84].
- The replacement and dialysate fluids should have the same composition to reduce staff confusion and the risk for error.
- CVVHDF requires the use of a blood, effluent, dialysate, and replacement pumps. Both dialysate and replacement solutions are used. Plasma water and solutes are removed by diffusion, convection, and ultrafiltration. In CVVHDF, removal of small molecules is achieved by diffusion through the addition of dialysate solution and removal of middle and large molecules by convection through addition of replacement solution. This transport mechanism is used only in CVVHDF.

- In adsorption, solute clearance takes place through molecular adherence to the surface of the membrane. This mechanism is used in SCUF, CVVH, CVVHD, and CVVHDF.
- CRRT clearance of solute is dependent on the molecule size of the solute, sieving coefficient, and the pore size of the semipermeable membrane. The higher the ultrafiltration rate, the greater the solute clearance. Small molecules easily pass through a membrane driven by diffusion and convection. Middle- and large-size molecules are cleared primarily by convection. The semipermeable membrane removes solutes with a molecular weight of up to 50,000 Da. Plasma proteins or substances that are highly protein bound will not be cleared.
- The sieving coefficient of a molecule is the ability of a substance to pass through a membrane from the blood compartment of the hemofilter to the fluid compartment. A sieving coefficient of 1 will allow the free passage of a substance; but a sieving coefficient of 0 indicates that the substance is unable to pass. The sieving coefficient of sodium is 0.94, potassium 1.0, creatinine 1.0, and albumin 0 [42–45, 93].
- It is recommended to continue CRRT as long as the criteria defining severe oliguric AKI are present. If the clinical condition improves, it may be considered to wait before connecting a new circuit to see whether renal function recovers. CRRT should be restarted in case of clinical or metabolic deterioration [5, 35–37, 94].
- CRRT may be postponed when the underlying disease is improving, other organ failure is recovering, and the slope in the serum creatinine rise declines, in order to see if renal function is also recovering.
- Establishing vascular access is a key factor for successful CRRT in children [4, 32, 78, 95]. The internal jugular vein is the primary site of choice due to a lower associated risk of complication and simplicity of catheter insertion. The femoral vein is optimal and constitutes the easiest site for insertion. The subclavian vein is the least preferred site given its higher risk of pneumonia/hemothorax and its association with central venous stenosis. The length of the catheter chosen will depend upon the site used. Two single-lumen venous hemodialysis catheters can be used in infants. Recommended catheters by age are <6 months, 4–5 F single lumen; 6–12 months, 5–7 F double lumen; 1–3 years, 8–9 F double lumen; and >3 years, 8–12 F double lumen [30, 31, 78].
- The semipermeable membrane is structurally designed to allow high fluid removal and molecular cutoff weight of 30,000–50,000 Da. The membrane provides an interface between the blood and dialysate compartment. The membrane biocompatibility minimizes severe patient reactions and decreases the complement activation [28, 29].
- Filters and tubing with a low prefilled volume should be used to reduce the blood volume in extracorporeal circulation and help ameliorate the decrease in effective circulating blood volume. Filters with a high-molecular-weight polymer membrane, high permeability, good biocompatibility, and small impact on the coagulation system should be selected. The use of AN69 membranes has been linked to bradykinin release syndrome among patients who are acidotic or taking

angiotensin-converting enzyme inhibitors [26, 29]. Alternative membranes should be used in such cases. Generally, the blood volume in extracorporeal circulation should be maintained at <10 % of body weight, e.g., <30 mL in neonates, <50 mL in infants, and <100 mL in children. For neonates weighing <2.5 kg, tubing can be prefilled with plasma, whole blood, or 5 % albumin.

- For continuous modes of renal replacement therapy to be effective, in terms of both effective solute clearance and also fluid removal, the extracorporeal circuits must operate continuously. Thus, preventing clotting in the CRRT circuit is a key goal to effective patient management. As these patients may also be at increased risk of bleeding, regional anticoagulation with citrate is increasing in popularity, particularly following the introduction of commercially available CRRT machines and fluids specifically designed for citrate anticoagulation. Although regional anticoagulation with citrate provides many advantages over other systemic anticoagulants, excess citrate may lead to metabolic complications, ranging from acidosis to alkalosis, and may also potentially expose patients to electrolyte disturbances due to hyper- and hyponatremia and hyper- and hypocalcemia.
- Transmembrane pressure should be monitored and maintained at <200 mmHg (note: a transmembrane pressure >250 mmHg may indicate clotting in the filter). Particular attention should be paid to warming the replacement fluid. The recommended flow rates are as follows: blood flow, 30 mL/min in neonates, 30–40 mL/min in infants/young children, 50–75 mL/min in children weighing <20 kg, and 75–100 mL/min in children weighing >20 kg; ultrafiltration rate, 8–10 mL/min/m^2 in neonates/infants and 8–15 mL/min/m^2 in children (note: daily fluid input/output, cardiac function, and edema should be considered); and dialysates, 15–20 mL/min/m^2 in neonates/infants/children [96].
- A simple and easy method for estimating drug clearance as a function of total creatinine clearance when the information on the pharmacokinetics of a particular drug is not available is to add replacement fluid rate (CVVH) or dialysate flow rate (CVVHD), usually 2 L/1.73 m^2/h or 33 mL/1.73 m^2/min, to the patient's native creatinine clearance (mL/1.73 m^2/min). This value is the patient's new creatinine clearance and dose drugs accordingly.
- Patients treated with continuous renal therapies in the ICU are probably at risk for antibiotic underdosing and therapeutic failures [28, 42, 51, 52, 59, 97–103].
- Estimation of renal function in acute injury is very challenging, but recently short-interval creatinine clearance measurements have been demonstrated.
- Widely available drug databases support individualized decision-making [102].
- There is little literature to support adjusting the loading dose of antibiotic in AKI.
- The sum of renal creatinine clearance and CVVH ultrafiltration provides a starting point for subsequent antibiotic dosing.
- When available, therapeutic drug monitoring should be used, especially for drugs with low therapeutic index.
- Loss of macro- and micronutrients is well documented during CRRT and, in general, requires replenishing or compensating eventual deficits [104–112].
- The final aim should be to optimize the nutritional status of the patient and to reduce the so-called dialytrauma induced by CRRT. Daily recommended energy

requirements during CRRT fluctuate between 25 and 35 kcal/kg (60–70 % carbohydrates and 30–40 % lipids) and between 1.5 and 1.8 g/kg protein. Significant alterations of carbohydrate and lipid metabolism as well as severe electrolyte disturbances may be found in patients undergoing CRRT. Close monitoring of these metabolic parameters and their interactions is imperative. Energy requirements during CRRT are increased and should best be assessed by indirect calorimetry. However, this technique is not universally available and will need correction for the known bicarbonate/CO_2 diversion induced by CRRT. The current ESPEN guidelines allow us to adequately supplement important micronutrients such as amino acids (glutamine), water-soluble vitamins, and trace elements. More widespread recognition of "dialytrauma" and the use of an appropriate checklist may help the bedside clinician to better assess and handle nutrition deficits in CRRT patients.

References

1. Auron A, Brophy PD. Pediatric renal supportive therapies: the changing face of pediatric renal replacement approaches. Curr Opin Pediatr. 2010;22:183–8.
2. Boschee ED, Cave DA, Garros D, Lequier L, Granoski DA, Guerra GG, et al. Indications and outcomes in children receiving renal replacement therapy in pediatric intensive care. J Crit Care. 2014;29:37–42.
3. Brophy PD, Maxvold NJ, Bunchman TE. CAVH/CVVH in pediatric patients. In: Nissenson AR, Fine RN, editors. Dialysis therapy. 3rd ed. Philadelphia: Hanley & Belfus; 2002.
4. Bunchman TE, Maxvold NJ, Kershaw DB, et al. Continuous veno-venous hemodiafiltration in infants and children. Pediatr Nephrol. 1994;8:96–9.
5. Burchardi H. Renal replacement therapy (RRT) in the ICU: criteria for initiating RRT. In: Ronco C, Bellomo R, La Greca G, editors. Blood purification in intensive care (Contributions to Nephrology V 132- Berlyne GM and Ronco C). New York: Karger; 2001. p. 171–80.
6. Clark WR, Mueller B, Kraus A, et al. Extracorporeal therapy requirements for patients with acute renal failure. J Am Soc Nephrol. 1997;8:804–12.
7. Elahi MM, Lim MY, Joseph RN, et al. Early hemofiltration improves survival in post-cardiotomy patients with acute renal failure. Eur J Cardiothorac Surg. 2004;26(5):1027–31.
8. Goldstein SL. Continuous renal replacement therapy: mechanism of clearance, fluid removal, indications and outcomes. Curr Opin Pediatr. 2011;23:181–5.
9. Goldstein SL, Somers MJ, Baum M, et al. Pediatric patients with multi-organ system failure receiving continuous renal replacement therapy. Kidney Int. 2005;67(2):653–8.
10. Naka T, Wan L, Bellomo R, et al. Kidney failure associated with liver transplantation or liver failure: the impact of continuous veno-venous hemofiltration. Int J Artif Organs. 2004;27(11): 949–55.
11. Silvester W. Mediator removal with CRRT: complement and cytokines. Am J Kidney Dis. 1997;30(5 Suppl 4):S38–43.
12. Zhang YL, Hu WP, Zhou LH, Wang Y, Cheng A, Shao SN, Hon LL, Chen QY. Continuous renal replacement therapy in children with multiple organ dysfunction syndrome: a case series. Int Braz J Urol. 2014;40(6):846–52.
13. Zobel G, Ring E, Rödl S. Prognosis in pediatric patients with multiple organ system failure and continuous extracorporeal renal support. Contrib Nephrol. 1995;116:163–8.
14. Askenazi DJ, Goldstein MD, Koralkar R, Fortenberry MD, Baum M, et al. Continuous renal replacement therapy for children ≤10 kg: a report from the prospective pediatric continuous renal replacement therapy registry. J Pediatr. 2013;162:587–92.

15. Gottlieb R, Assadi F. Continuous renal replacement therapy in newborn infants. In: Spitzer AR, editor. Intensive care of the fetus and neonate. Philadelphia: Mosby-Year Book; 1995. p. 1187–91.
16. Ronco C, Garzotto F, Brendolan A, Zanella M, Bellettato M, Vedovato S, et al. Continuous renal replacement therapy in neonates and small infants: development and use of a miniaturised machine (CARPEDIEM). Lancet. 2014;383(9931):1807–13.
17. Sohn YB, Paik KH, Cho HY, Kim SJ, Park SW, Kim ES, et al. Continuous renal replacement therapy in neonates weighing less than 3 kg. Korean J Pediatr. 2012;55(8):286–92.
18. Symons JM, Brophy PD, Gregory MJ, et al. Continuous renal replacement therapy in children up to 10 kg. Am J Kidney Dis. 2003;41(5):984–9.
19. Bunchman TE. Fluid overload in multiple organ dysfunction syndrome: a prediction of survival. Crit Care Med. 2004;32(8):1805–6.
20. Foland JA, Fortenberry JD, Warshaw BL, et al. Fluid over load before continuous hemofiltration and survival in critically ill children: a retrospective analysis. Crit Care Med. 2004;32(8):1771–6.
21. Gillespie RS, Seidel K, Symons JM. Effect of fluid overload and dose of replacement fluid on survival in hemofiltration. Pediatr Nephrol. 2004;19(12):1394–9.
22. Goldstein SL. Overview of pediatric renal replacement therapy in acute kidney injury. Semin Dial. 2009;22:180–4.
23. Mehta RL, Clark WC, Schetz M. Techniques for assessing and achieving fluid balance in acute renal failure. Curr Opin Crit Care. 2002;8:535–43.
24. Piccinni P, Dan M, Barbacini S, et al. Early isovolaemic haemofiltration in oliguric patients with septic shock. Intensive Care Med. 2006;32(1):80–6.
25. Sutherland SM, Zappitelli M, Alexander SR, Chua AN, Brophy PD, Bunchman TE, et al. Fluid overload and mortality in children receiving continuous renal replacement therapy: the prospective pediatric continuous renal replacement therapy registry. Am J Kidney Dis. 2010;55(2):316–25.
26. Baird JS, Wald EL. Long-term (>4wels) continuous renal replacement therapy in critical illness. Int J Artif Organs. 2010;33(10):716–20.
27. Lopez-Herce J, Santiago MJ, Solana MJ, Urbano J, del Castillo J, Carrillo A, et al. Clinical course of children requiring prolonged continuous renal replacement therapy. Pediatr Nephrol. 2010;25(3):523–8.
28. Brophy PD, Mottes TA, Kudelka TL, et al. AN-69 membrane reactions are pH-dependent and preventable. Am J Kidney Dis. 2001;38(1):173–8.
29. McDonald BR, Mehta RL. Transmembrane flux of IL-1B and TNF-alpha in patients undergoing continuous arteriovenous hemodialysis (CAVHD). J Am Soc Nephrol. 1990;1:368–71.
30. Bambauer R, Inniger R, Pirrung KJ, et al. Complications and side effects associated with large-bore catheters in the subclavian and internal jugular veins. Artif Organs. 1994;18:318–21.
31. Cimochowski GE, Worley E, Rutherford WE, et al. Superiority of the internal jugular over the subclavian access for temporary dialysis. Nephron. 1990;54:154–61.
32. Hackbarth R, Bunchman TE, Chue AN, et al. The effect of vascular access location and size on circuit survival in pediatric continuous renal support therapy: a report from the PCRRT registry. Int J Artif Organs. 2007;30:1116–21.
33. Jenkins RD, Kuhn RJ, Funk JE. Clinical implications of catheter variability on neonatal continuous hemofiltration. Trans Am Soc Artif Intern Organs. 1998;34:108–11.
34. McBryde KD, Bunchman TE, Kudelka TL, et al. Hyperosmolar solutions in continuous renal replacement therapy for hyperosmolar acute renal failure: a preliminary report. Pediatr Crit Care Med. 2005;6(2):228–39.
35. Kim HJ, Park SL, Park KI, Lee JS, Eun HS, Kim JH, et al. Acute treatment of hyperammonemia by continuous renal replacement therapy in a newborn patient with ornithine transcarbamylase deficiency. Korean J Pediatr. 2011;54(10):425–8.
36. Deodato F, Boenzi S, Rizzo C, et al. Inborn errors of metabolism: an update on epidemiology and on neonatal-onset hyperammonemia. Acta Paediatr Suppl. 2004;93(445):18–21.
37. McBryde KD, Kershaw DB, Bunchman TE, et al. Renal replacement therapy in the treatment of confirmed or suspected inborn errors of metabolism. J Pediatr. 2006;148(6):770–8.

38. Ronco C, Ricci Z. Pediatric continuous renal replacement: 20 years later. Intensive Care Med. 2015;41(6):985–93.
39. Gibney N, Hoste E, Burdmann EA, Bunchman T, Kher V, Viswanathan R, et al. Timing of initiation and discontinuation of renal replacement therapy in AKI: unanswered key questions. Clin J Am Soc Nephrol. 2008;3:876–80.
40. Paganini E, O'Hara P, Nakamoto S. Slow continuous ultrafiltration in hemodialysis resistant oliguric renal failure. Trans Am Soc Artif Intern Organs. 1984;30:173–8.
41. Parakininkas D, Greenbaum LA. Comparison of solute clearance in three modes of continuous renal replacement therapy. Pediatr Crit Care Med. 2004;5(3):269–74.
42. Bauer SR, Salem C, Connor Jr MJ, Groszek J, Taylor ME, Wei P, Tolwani AJ, Fissell WH. Pharmacokinetics and pharmacodynamics of piperacillin-tazobactam in 42 patients treated with concomitant CRRT. Clin J Am Soc Nephrol. 2012;7(3):452–7.
43. Bugge JF. Pharmacokinetics and drug dosing adjustments during continuous venovenous hemofiltration or hemodiafiltration in critically ill patients. Acta Anaesthesiol Scand. 2001;45(8):929–34.
44. Kuang D, Verbine A, Ronco C. Pharmacokinetics and antimicrobial dosing adjustment in critically ill patients during continuous renal replacement therapy. Clin Nephrol. 2007;67:267–84.
45. Lau AH, Kronfol NO. Determinants of drug removal by continuous hemofiltration. Int J Artif Organs. 1994;17:373–8.
46. Taylor CA, Abdel-Rahman E, Zimmerman SW, Johnson CA. Clinical pharmacokinetics during continuous ambulatory peritoneal dialysis. Clin Pharmacokinet. 1996;31:293–308.
47. Varghese JM, Jarrett P, Boots RJ, Kirkpatrick CM, Lipman J, Roberts J. Pharmacokinetics of piperacillin and tazobactam in plasma and subcutaneous interstitial fluid in critically ill patients receiving continuous venovenous haemodiafiltration. Int J Antimicrob Agents. 2014;43:343–48.
48. Vincent HH, Vos MC, Akcahuseyin E, Goessens WH, van Duyl WA, Schalekamp MA. Drug clearance by continuous haemodiafiltration: analysis of sieving coefficients and mass transfer coefficients of diffusion. Blood Purif. 1993;11:99–107.
49. Vos MC, Vincent HH, Yzerman EPF, Vogel M, Mouton JW. Drug clearance by continuous haemodiafiltration: results with the AN-69 capillary haemofilter and recommended dose adjustment for seven antibiotics. Drug Invest. 1994;7:315–22.
50. Buckmaster JN, Davis AR. Guidelines for drug dosing during continuous renal replacement therapies. In: Ronco C, Bellomo R, editors. Critical care nephrology. Heidelberg: Springer; 1998. p. 1327–34.
51. Carcelero E, Soy D. Antibiotic dose adjustment in the treatment of MRSA infections in patients with acute renal failure undergoing continuous renal replacement therapies. Enferm Infect Microbiol Clin. 2012;30(5):249–56.
52. Choi G, Gomersall CD, Tian Q, Joynt GM, Freebairn R, Lipman J. Principal of antibacterial dosing in continuous renal replacement therapy. Blood Purif. 2010;30:195–212.
53. Covajes C, Scolletta S, Penaccini L, Ocampos-Martinez E, Abdelhadii A, Beumier M, Jacobs F, de Backer D, Vincent JL, Taccone FS. Continuous infusion of vancomycin in septic patients receiving continuous renal replacement therapy. Int J Antimicrob Agents. 2013;41:261–6.
54. Choi G, Gomersall CD, Tian Q, Joynt GM, Freebairn R, Lipman J. Principles of antibacterial dosing in continuous renal replacement therapy. Crit Care Med. 2009;37:2268–82.
55. Li AM, Gomersall CD, Choi G, Tian Q, Joynt GM, Lipman J. A systematic review of antibiotic dosing regimens for septic patients receiving continuous renal replacement therapy: do current studies supply sufficient data? J Antimicrob Chemother. 2009;64:929–37.
56. Mattzke GR, Aronoff GR, Atkinson Jr AJ, et al. Drug dosing consideration in patients with acute and chronic kidney disease: a clinical update from kidney disease: improving global outcomes (KDIGO). Kidney Int. 2011;80:1120–37.
57. Reetze-Bonorden P, Böhler J, Keller E. Drug dosage in patients during continuous renal replacement therapy: pharmacokinetic and therapeutic considerations. Clin Pharmacokinet. 1993;24:362–79.
58. Subach RA, Marx MA. Drug dosing in acute renal failure: the role of renal replacement therapy in altering drug pharmacokinetics. Adv Ren Replace Ther. 1998;5:141–7.

59. Veltri MA, Neu AM, Fivush BA, Parekh RS, Furth SL. Drug dosing during intermittent hemodialysis and continuous renal replacement therapy: special considerations in pediatric patients. Pediatr Drugs. 2004;6:45–65.
60. Lameire N, Van Biesen W, Vanholder R. Electrolyte disturbances and acute kidney injury in patients with cancer. Semin Nephrol. 2010;30:534–47.
61. Macias WA, Clark WR. Acid base balance in continuous renal replacement therapy. Semin Dial. 1996;9:145–51.
62. Assadi F. Strategies to reduce the incident of chronic kidney disease in children: time to change. J Nephrol. 2012;26:41–7.
63. Goldstein SL, Devarajan P. Acute kidney injury leads to pediatric patient mortality. Nat Rev Nephrol. 2010;6:393–4.
64. Bagshaw SM. Epidemiology of renal recovery after acute renal failure. Curr Opin Crit Care. 2006;12(6):544–50.
65. Bunchman TE, McBryde KD, Mottes TE, et al. Pediatric acute renal failure: outcome by modality and disease. Pediatr Nephrol. 2001;16(12):1067–71.
66. Coca SG, Yusuf B, Shlipak MG, et al. Long-term risk of mortality and other adverse outcomes after acute kidney injury: a systematic review and meta-analysis. Am J Kidney Dis. 2009;53:961–73.
67. Hui-Stickle S, Brewer ED, Goldstein SL. Pediatric ARF epidemiology at a tertiary care center from 1999 to 2001. Am J Kidney Dis. 2005;45:96–101.
68. Waikar SS, Liu KD, Chertow GM. Diagnosis, epidemiology and outcomes of acute kidney injury. Clin J Am Soc Nephrol. 2008;3:844–61.
69. Akcan-Arikan A, Zappitelli M, Loftis LL, Washburn KK, Jefferson LS, Goldstein SL. Modified RIFLE criteria in critically ill children with acute kidney injury. Kidney Int. 2007;71:1028–35.
70. Roy AK, Mc Gorrian C, Treacy C, Kavanaugh E, Brenner A, Mahon NG, et al. A comparison of traditional and novel definition (RIFLE, AKIN, and KDIGO) of acute kidney injury for the prediction of outcomes in acute decompensated heart failure. Cardiorenal Med. 2013;3(1):26–37.
71. Argyri I, Xanthos T, Varsami M, Aroni F, Papalois A, Dontas I, et al. The role of novel biomarkers in early diagnosis of acute kidney injury in newborns. Am J Perinatol. 2013;30:347–52.
72. Coca SG, Yalavarthy R, Concato J, Parikh CR. Biomarkers for the diagnosis and risk stratification of acute kidney injury: a systematic review. Kidney Int. 2008;73:1008–16.
73. Devarajan P. Emerging urinary biomarkers in the diagnosis of acute kidney injury. Expert Opin Med Diagn. 2008;2:387–98.
74. Han WK, Waiker SS, Johnson A, Betensky RA, Dent CL, Devarajan P, et al. Urinary biomarkers in the early detection of acute kidney injury. Kidney Int. 2008;73(7):863–9.
75. Liangos O, Tighiouart H, Perianayagam MC, Kolyada A, Han WK, Wald R, et al. Comparative analysis of urinary biomarkers for early detection of acute kidney injury following cardiopulmonary bypass. Biomarkers. 2009;14(6):423–32.
76. Fleming GM, Walters S, Goldstein SL, Alexander SR, Baum MA, Blowey DL, et al. Nonrenal indications for continuous renal replacement therapy: a report from the prospective pediatric continuous renal replacement therapy registry group. Pediatr Crit Care Med. 2012;13:e299–304.
77. Korneckki A, Tauman R, Lubetzky R, Sivan Y. Continuous renal replacement therapy for non-renal indications: experience in children. Isr Med Assoc J. 2002;4(5):345–8.
78. Bunchman TE. Wilson SE (eds) Vascular access: principles and practice. 4th ed. St. Louis: Mosby; 2002. Pediatr Nephrol. 2003;18(9):968.
79. Goonasekera CD, Wang J, Bunchman TE, Deep A. Factors affecting circuit life during continuous renal replacement therapy in children with liver failure. Ther Apher Dial. 2015;19(1):16–22.
80. Ricci Z, Guzzo I, Picca S, Picardo S. Circuit lifespan during continuous renal replacement therapy: children and adults are not equal. Crit Care. 2008;12(5):178.
81. Barenbrock M, Hausberg M, Marzkies F, et al. Effects of bicarbonate- and lactate- buffered replacement fluids on cardiovascular outcome in CVVH patients. Kidney Int. 2000;58:1751–7.

82. Bunchman TE, Maxvold NJ, Barnett J, et al. Pediatric hemofiltration: Normocarb® dialysate solution with citrate anticoagulation. Pediatr Nephrol. 2002;17:150–4.
83. Bunchman TE, Maxvold NJ, Brophy PD. Pediatric convective hemofiltration: Normocarb® replacement fluid and citrate anticoagulation. Am J Kidney Dis. 2003;42(6):1248–52.
84. Levraut J, Ciebiera JP, Jambou P, et al. Effect of continuous venovenous hemofiltration with dialysis on lactate clearance in critically ill patients. Crit Care Med. 1997;25:58–62.
85. Roy D, Hogg RJ, Wilby PA, et al. Continuous veno-venous hemodiafiltration using bicarbonate dialysate. Pediatr Nephrol. 1997;11(6):680–3.
86. Tobe SW, Murphy PM, Goldberg P, et al. A new sterile bicarbonate dialysis solution for use during cardiopulmonary bypass. ASAIO J. 1999;45(3):157–9.
87. Zimmerman D, Cotman P, Ting R, et al. Continuous veno-venous haemodialysis with a novel bicarbonate dialysis solution: prospective cross-over comparison with a lactate buffered solution. Nephrol Dial Transplant. 1999;14:2387–91.
88. Bellomo R. Choosing a therapeutic modality: hemofiltration vs. hemodialysis vs. hemodiafiltration. Semin Dial. 1996;9:88–92.
89. Brophy PD, Somers MJ, Baum MA, et al. Multicenter evaluation of anticoagulation in patients receiving continuous renal replacement therapy (CRRT). Nephrol Dial Transplant. 2005;20(7):1416–21.
90. Flynn JT. Choice of dialysis modality for management of pediatric acute renal failure. Pediatr Nephrol. 2002;17:61–9. AKI REVIEW.
91. Jiang HL, Xue WJ, Li DQ, et al. Pre- vs. post-dilution CVVH. Blood Purif. 2005;23(4):338.
92. Ronco C, Belomo R, Homel P, et al. Effects of different doses in continuous venovenous hemofiltration on outcomes of acute renal failure: a prospective randomized trial. Lancet. 2000;356:26–30.
93. Bressolle F, Kinowski JM, de la Coussaye JE, Wynn N, Eledjam JJ, Galtier M. Clinical pharmacokinetics during continuous haemofiltration. Clin Pharmacokinet. 1994;26:457–71.
94. Picca S, Dionisi-Vici C, Abeni D, et al. Extracorporeal dialysis in neonatal hyperammonemia: modalities and prognostic indicators. Pediatr Nephrol. 2001;16(11):862–7.
95. Bunchman TE, Gardner JJ, Kershaw DB, Maxvold NJ. Vascular access for hemodialysis or CVVH(D) in infants and children. Nephrol Dial Transplant. 1994;23:314–7.
96. Webb AR, Mythen MG, Jacobson D, et al. Maintaining blood flow in the extracorporeal circuit. Intensive Care Med. 1995;21:84–93.
97. Bareletta JF, Barletta GM, Brophy PD, Maxvold NJ, Hackbarth RM, Bunchman TE. Medication errors and patient complications with continuous renal replacement therapy. Pediatr Nephrol. 2006;21:842–5.
98. Bunchman TE. Medication errors and patient complications with continuous renal replacement therapy. Pediatr Nephrol. 2006;21:842–5.
99. Churchwell MD, Mueller BA. Drug dosing during continuous renal replacement therapy. Semin Dial. 2009;22(2):185–8.
100. Connor Jr MJ, Salem C, Bauer SR, Hofmann CL, Groszek J, Butler R, Rehm SJ, Fissell WH. Therapeutic drug monitoring of piperacillin-tazobactam using spent dialysate effluent in patients receiving continuous venovenous hemodialysis. Antimicrob Agents Chemother. 2011;55:557–60.
101. Jamal JA, Economou CJ, Lipman J, Roberts JA. Improving antibiotic dosing in special situations in the ICU: burns, renal replacement therapy and extracorporeal membrane oxygenation. Curr Opin Crit Care. 2012;18:460–71.
102. Keller F, Böhler J, Czock D, Zellner D, Mertz AKH. Individualized drug dosage in patients treated with continuous hemofiltration. Kidney Int. 1999;56 Suppl 72:S29–31.
103. Roder BL, Frimodt-Moller N, Espersen F, Rasmussen SN. Dicloxacillin and flucloxacillin: pharmacokinetics, protein binding and serum bactericidal titers in healthy subjects after oral administration. Infection. 1995;23:107–12.
104. Campbell IT. Limitations of nutrient intake: the effect of stressors: trauma, sepsis and multiple organ failure. Eur J Clin Nutr. 1999;53 Suppl 1:S143–7.

105. Castillo A, Santiago MJ, Lopez-Hirce J, Montoro S, Lopez J, Bustinza A, et al. Nutritional status and clinical outcome of children on continuous renal replacement therapy: a prospective observational study. BMC Nephrol. 2012;13:125.
106. Davies SP, Reaveley DA, Brown EA, Kox WJ. Amino acid clearance and daily losses in patients with acute renal failure treated by continuous arteriovenous hemodialysis. Crit Care Med. 1991;19(12):1510–5.
107. Hmiel SP, Martin RA, Landt M, et al. Amino acid clearance during acute metabolic decompensation in maple syrup urine disease treated with continuous venovenous hemodialysis with filtration. Pediatr Crit Care Med. 2004;5(3):278–81.
108. Maxvold NJ, Smoyer WE, Custer JR, Bunchman TE. Amino acid loss and nitrogen balance in critically ill children with acute renal failure: a comparison between CVVH and CVVHD therapies. Crit Care Med. 2000;28:1161–5.
109. McBryde KD, Kudelka TL, Kershaw DB, et al. Clearance of amino acids by hemodialysis in argininosuccinate synthetase deficiency. J Pediatr. 2004;144(4):536–40.
110. Meyer TW, Walther JL, Pagtalunan ME, et al. The clearance of protein bound solutes by hemofiltration and hemodiafiltration. Kidney Int. 2005;68(2):867–77.
111. Zappiteli M, Seymons JM, Somers MJG, et al. Protein and caloric intake prescription of children receiving continuous renal support therapy: a report from the prospective pediatric continuous renal support therapy registry group. Pediatr Crit Care Med. 2008;36:3239–45.
112. Zappitelli M, Juarez M, Castillo L, Cross-Bu J, Gildstein SL. Continuous renal replacement therapy amino acid, trace element, and folate clearance in critically ill children. Intensive Care Med. 2009;35:698–706.

Appendix

F. Assadi, F.G. Sharbaf, *Pediatric Continuous Renal Replacement Therapy*,
DOI 10.1007/978-3-319-26202-4

CRRT Order Sheet

Date___________________

Time_____________

Hemofiltration Day #________

Patient Weight (kg)_______________

Patient Surface Area (1.73M^2)_____________

Allergies____

Type of Modality:

- ❑ SCUF (Slow Continuous Ultrafiltration)
- ❑ CVVH with replacement fluid
- ❑ CVVHD with dialysate
- ❑ CVVHDF with both replacement fluid and dialysate

Filter:

- □ M60 (0.6 m^2): Total extracorporeal blood volume of 93 $\pm$ 10% ml ($\leq$50 Kg)
- □ M100 (0.9 m^2): Total extracorporeal blood volume of 152 $\pm$ 10% ml (>50 Kg)

Priming:

❑ Normal Saline	❑ NS with 5000 units heparin in 1000 ml normal saline	❑ Blood Prime See Protocol

*If machine is not used within 15 minutes of prime, re-prime with at least 500ml of prime solution

Blood Flow Rate (Q_B): _________ ml/min (standard rate 4-5 ml/kg/min). Minimum Q_B 50 ml/min for M60 and 75 ml/.min for M100 (Optimal rate: 100-200 ml/min)

Patient Fluid Removal Rate: ________ ml/hr (recommended net loss 1-2 ml/kg/hr)

Dialysate Rate; ____________________mL/hr (recommended 2000 mL/1.73m^2/hr)

ACD-A Rate: ____________________mL/hr (start at 1.5 x BFR)

Calcium Chloride Rate: _____________mL/hr (start at 0.4 x ACD-A rate)

Titrate calcium chloride infusion to maintain patient ionized calcium between 1.1-1.3 (Table 15).

Titrate ACD-A infusion rate to maintain PRISMA ionized calcium between) 0.25-0.35 (Table 14).

Heparin dose adjustment

To determine heparin concentration as follow:

Patient weight	Heparin concentration*
<10 kg	40 units/ml
11-25 kg	100 units/ml
16-60 kg	250 units/ml
>60 kg	500 units/ml

* PRISMA heparin rate must be >0.5 ml/hr.

Initial bolus 20 units/Kg (administer pre-filter). Subsequent hourly continuous infusion (10-20 units/kg/hr) is given to maintain APTT of 1.5 to 2.5 times the control value (25-35 seconds).

Adjust heparin infusion rate according to APTT as follow

APTT (seconds)	Heparin infusion rate
50-80	**No Change**
<50	Bolus by 10 units/kg, increase by 10% and recheck APPT in one hour
>80	Hold heparin infusion by ½ hour, decrease by 10% and recheck APPT in one hour

Anticoagulation:

❑ Heparin ------------- units/ml in 20ml syringe Deliver on heparin syringe line Loading dose: (20u/kg)__________ _ Continuous	❑ *Citrate (ACD-A) Starting rate: 1.5 x BFR_______ml/hr Deliver on white scale (PBP scale). Must use systemic on the pre-filter of the hemofiltration access	❑ *Calcium Chloride: 8.0 g in 1000 ml 0.9% saline Starting rate: 0.4 x ACD-A_____ ml/hr Deliver via IV pump on return line

infusion rate (5-20u/kg)____u/kg/hr

ACT	Heparin adjustment
<170	10-20u/kg bolus and Increase dose by 10% and recheck ACT 1hr
170-220	No change
>220	Hold heparin for 1hr, then restart at 10% reduced

Post-filter ionized calcium (mmol/L)	Citrate adjustment
<0.25	Decrease by 5 ml/hr
0.25-0.39	No change
0.40-0.50	Increase by 5 ml/hr
>0.5	Increase by 10 ml/hr

* Must order calcium chloride infusion

Systemic ionized calcium (mmol/L)	Calcium chloride adjustment
>1.3	Decrease by 10ml/hr
1.1-1.3	No change
0.9-1.1	Increase by 10 ml/hr
<0.9	Increase by 20 ml/hr
<0.9 or >1.3	Call Nephrologist

* Must order citrate infusion

		dose and recheck ACT 1hr		

Dialysate (Green Scale): (for use with CVVHD or CVVHDF only). **Dialysate Rate** ml/min, starting rate: 500 ml/1.73m^2/hr (recommended 2000 ml/1.73 m^2/hr)

• **Commercial Solutions:**

Bicarbonate- based (mEq/L)	Na^+	K^+	Cl^-	$HCO3^-$	Ca^{++}	Mg^{++}	Glucose (mg/dl)	lactate	Osmolality (mOsm/L)
❑ BK0/3.5	140	0	109	32	3.5	1.0	0	3	287
❑ BGK2/0	140	0	108	32	0	1.0	110	3	292
❑ BGK4/0	140	4	110	32	0	1.5	110	3	296
❑ BGK4/2.5	140	4	113	32	2.5	1.5	110	3	300
❑ B25GK4/0	140	4	120	22	0	1.5	110	3	296
❑ BK2/0	140	2	108	32	0	1.0	0	3	286

Lactate-based

- Dianeal 1.5% 132 0 96 0 3.5

  0.5 1500 40 347

- Baxter Hemofilter (HF) 140 2 117 0 1.5

  1.0 100 30 285

•Custom Dialysate

- **Calcium Solution**

  NaCl_______(100 mEq/L)

  $NaHCO3^-$ ______(40 mEq/L)

  KCl_______(4 mEq/L)

  MgSO4_____(0.5-1.5 mEq/L)

  $CaCl^2$_______(3.5 mEq/L)

  Dextrose_______ 1.5g/L

- **Phosphorus Solutior**

  NaCl _____ 100 (mEq/L)

  $NaHCO3^-$ _____(40 mEq/L)

  KCl _____(2mEq/L)

  MgSO4_____(0.5-1.5 mEq/L)

  K3PO4_____(2 mEq/L)

  Dextrose _____(1.5 g/L)

Replacement: (for use with CVVH or CVVHDF only).

Replacement Rate:__________ml/hr (off or 100-1500 ml/1.73m^2/hr). Starting rate: 200 ml/hr

☐ BK0/3.5 ☐ BGK2/0 ☐ BGK4/0 ☐ BGK4/2.5 ☐ B25GK4/0

☐ BK2/0 ☐ Dianeal 1.5% ☐ Baxter HF ☐ Additives___________

Replacement Delivery Method:

- ❑ 100% pre dilution CVVH or CVVHDF Place replacement on purple scale
- ❑ 100% post dilution CVVH or CVVHDF Place replacement on purple scale
- ❑ Pre and Post dilution CVVH only
  - ❑ _____% pre (purple scale)
  - ❑ _____% post (green scale)

Lab Tests:

- ❑ ACT: Hourly for 2-3 hours, then every 4 hours
- ❑ Post-filter ionized calcium and CBC: At initiation, then every six hours
- ❑ Systemic ionized calcium: At initiation, then every six hours
- ❑ Renal Panel with magnesium, phosphorous, HB/HCT: At initiation, then every 12 hours

Physician Signature/Date______________________________

Dialysis Nurse Signature/Date______________________________

Electrolytes Replacement Protocol

Calcium Chloride (Ca^{++}) Infusion (to be used with Phosphorous solutions only). Add calcium chloride 8.0 g in 1000 ml of 0.9% NaCl **(infuse in central line other than hemofiltration access).**

Infusion rate ____________ (5 mg/kg/hr administer via central line ONLY)

Monitor systemic ionized calcium level (from prisma pre-filter) hourly until stable and then q 6 hours to adjust calcium infusion. Titrate $cacl_2$ infusion to maintain patient Ca^{++} of 1.1-1.3 mmol/l (2.2-2.6 mg/dl) below:

Patients Ca^{++} (mmol/L)	Ca^{++} infusion adjustment*
>1.3	Decrease rate by 10 ml/hr
1.1-1.3 (optimum range)	No adjustment
0.9-1.0	Increase rate by 10 ml/hr
<0.9	Increase rate by 20 ml/hr
<0.8 or >1.3	Call nephrologists

*Notify MD if patient Ca^{++} <1 or if rate requires changes 2 times in 12 hours

*Notify MD if calcium infusion rate >150 ml/hr

Magnesium (Mg^{++}) replacement*

Serum Mg^{++} level (mg/dL)	Mg^{++} dose (1.0 g/100 mlL5%DW)
0.5-0.9	1.0 g/hr x 3 dose
1.0-1.5	1.0 g/hr x 2 doses

<0.5 or >2.5	Call nephrologists

*Repeat Mg^{++} level 2 hours post-infusion

Sodium Phosphate ($PO4^-$) replacement*

Serum $PO4^-$ level (mg/dl)	Sodium $PO4^-$ dose (mM/100 ml 5%DW)
1.5-1.9	30 mM (infuse at 10 mM/hr)
2.0-2.5	20 mM (infuse at 10 mM/hr)
<1.5 or >5.0	Call nephrologist

*Repeat serum PO4 level 2 hours post-infusion

Potassium replacement (mEq/L)*

Serum K^+ level (mEq/L)	KCL dose
3.2-3.5	20 mEq/hr X 3 doses
3.6-3.9	20 mEq/hr x 2 doses
4.0-4.2	20 mEq/hr x1 and 10 mEq/hr x1
4.3-4.5	20 mEq/hr x 1 dose
<3.5 or>5.5	Call nephrologist

Repeat K^+ level 2 hours post-infusion

Vascular Access:

Weight (Kg)	Size	Access
3-15	Dual lumen 7.0 Fr dual lumen	UVC, Femoral, SC
16-30	9.0 Fr dual lumen	Femoral, SC, IJ
>30	11 Fr dual lumen	Femoral, SC, IJ

Index

F. Assadi, F.G. Sharbaf, *Pediatric Continuous Renal Replacement Therapy*,
DOI 10.1007/978-3-319-26202-4

Printed in the United States
By Bookmasters